Excitable Cells

Excitable Cells

F. A. Miles

Lecturer in Biology,
The University of Sussex.

William Heinemann Medical Books Limited
London

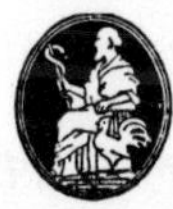

First published 1969
Reprinted 1979

S.B.N. 433 21971 8

For Jennifer

Printed in Hong Kong by Bright Sun Printing Press Co. Ltd

CONTENTS

PREFACE

The main concern of this book is with the fundamental nature of the signals carried about the nervous system. In historical terms, most of the evidence considered here (if not the ideas) is of recent origin and has been culled from work published in the last two decades. Little of this material has so far found its way into the traditional biological literature at either school or undergraduate levels. Whilst the important developments in this field have been well documented for the research worker and advanced student, few sources make concessions to the uninitiated and, essentially, I have attempted to reshape this material to give it more universal currency. This is especially true of the illustrations, many of which are based on figures taken from the original papers. I have been conscious of the need to impose some measure of standardization in presenting this evidence and have risked incurring the odium of the purists in adhering to this principle.

For permission to use illustrations, I am indebted to the authors cited in the legends and to the following publishers and editors of Journals:

Academic Press Inc., New York
Journal of Ultrastructure Research.
American Physiological Society, Bethesda, Md.
Journal of Neurophysiology.
Long Island Biological Association Inc., Cold Spring Harbor
Cold Spring Harbor Symposia on Quantitative Biology.
The Physiological Society, London
Journal of Physiology.
The Rockefeller University Press, New York
Journal of General Physiology.
The Royal Society of London, London
Proceedings.
The Scandinavian Society for Physiology, Stockholm
Acta physiologica scandinavica.
The Liverpool University Press, Liverpool
Conduction of the Nervous Impulse. A. L. Hodgkin.
The Hafner Publishing Co., New York and Methuen & Co. Ltd. London,
The Organisation of the Cerebral Cortex. D. A. Sholl.

It is a pleasure to thank Dr. C. Kidd for his comments on an early draft, Miss M. Waldron for most of the drawings and Mr. C. Atherton for invaluable photographic assistance. Finally, I should like to record my appreciation to my publishers and, in particular, to Dr. Catherine Clegg and Mr. Owen R. Evans for their ready cooperation and patient endeavours on technical matters.

F. A. MILES

May 1969.

CHAPTER 1

Elements of Structure and Function in the Nervous System

The brain of man is the most sophisticated achievement of evolution. Weighing only a few pounds, it encompasses a wealth of conducting units organized into networks of exquisite complexity. This central computer system is in continuous receipt of messages generated by peripheral sense organs which describe conditions in the environment. These input signals are carefully sifted and processed in the intricate networks of the central nervous system and any disturbing features which emerge from this analysis result in command signals being sent out to the executive organs, the muscles, to initiate counter-action. Even trivial mechanical operations such as holding this book call upon the nervous system to organize and coordinate the activity of numerous muscles. In so doing, a level of fluency and versatility is achieved which goes far beyond the capabilities of any control system devised by the engineer. It is this organization which enables man and animals to become aware of their surroundings, avoid the harmful and seek out food and refuge.

Recent developments in the applied sciences, particularly in electronics, have provided instruments with which the neurophysiologist can probe the workings of the individual units of this system. As a result, a great deal is now known about the signals which flow along the communication channnels of the body. The main concern of this book is with the fundamental nature of these signals and the ways in which they are generated and handled by the nervous system.

The Neurone

The neurones compose the elementary units of the nervous system, contriving immense variation of size and geometrical form whilst retaining certain features which are common to all such cells. Invariably the cell body, or soma, is invested by a delicate lipoprotein membrane which is thrust out into slender, irregular processes—the dendrites and the axon. The dendrites branch freely and insinuate themselves amongst the cell bodies and processes of other surrounding neurones. The single axon extends

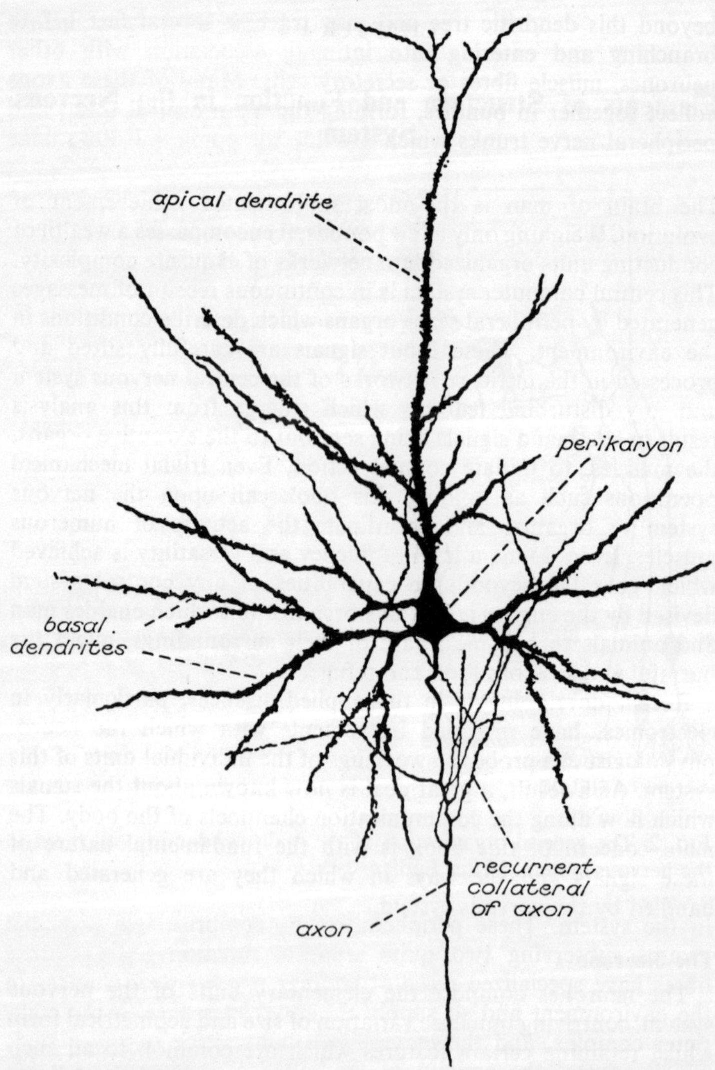

FIG. 1. A drawing of a pyramidal neurone from the cortex of a cat. The dendrites project in all directions and it is not possible to focus them all in one photograph. This drawing was made from a tracing of three photographs taken with the microscope focussed at different depths of a Golgi preparation. (Sholl, 1956.)

beyond this dendritic tree and may traverse several feet before branching and entering into intimate association with other neurones, muscle fibres or secretory cells. Many of these axons collect together in bundles, forming the main central tracts and peripheral nerve trunks which provide the communicating links

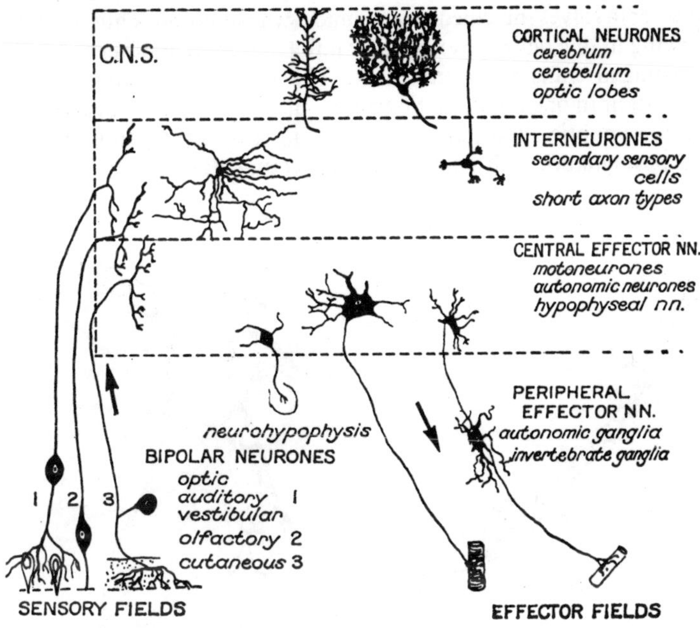

FIG. 2. The general organization of the main conducting cell types in the nervous system. (After Bodian, 1952.)

in the system. These peripheral axons comprise two principal groups subserving two quite separate functions: the *sensory* fibres have specialized receptor endings which signal changes in the environment and so supply the input messages to the computer complex, and the *motor* fibres convey the output signals which control the activity of the muscles and other excitable tissues.

The Synapse

Communication between neurones occurs only at special sites, the synapses, at each of which a swollen axon terminal from one cell abuts on to the cell body or dendrites of another. A narrow gap, less than a millionth of an inch across, separates the two neurones at the synapse and constitutes a definite break in the transmission line. The electrical signals carried about the nervous system are confined to the cells and transfer from one neurone to another involves intermediary chemical transmission. Thus, signals arriving in one neurone exert their influence upon another through a chemical transmitter substance. The information transfer can only occur in one direction however—the transmitter is released by the *pre*synaptic axon terminals, diffusing across the gap to act on the *post*synaptic cell body. The projecting dendrites provide a

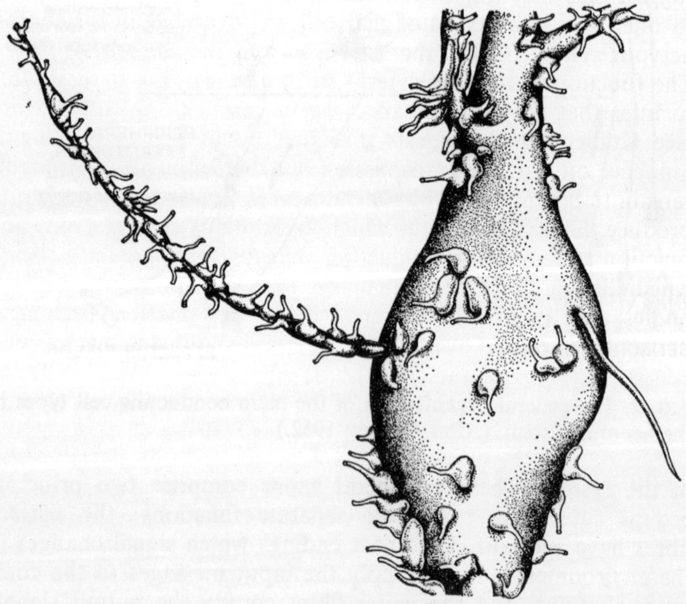

FIG. 3. A three-dimensional reconstruction of a neurone from the lateral geniculate nucleus of a rat. This is based upon serial sections studied under the electron microscope. Note the tendency for the synaptic endings on this particular neurone to cluster round the various processes. (Karlsson, 1966.)

generous extension of the soma membrane which enables the cell to accept incoming signals from large numbers of axon terminals. In a recent study of the surface layers of the brain using an electron microscope, Cragg (1967) estimates that some cells receive up to 60,000 terminals! The soma-dendritic membrane thus serves as the receiving area for the cell, where numerous converging signals are sorted and fashioned into an output message which is relayed down the axon to the next synapse.

The Neuroglial Cell

All neurones are in close association with non-conducting neuroglial cells. Although much smaller than neurones, these supporting cells probably take up about a half of the volume of the brain since they are far more numerous. Some authors suggest that they might outnumber neurones by as much as ten to one. Two main types of glial cell are identified in the central nervous system (CNS), the astrocytes and the oligodendrocytes. The function of the astrocytes is still polemical, but it seems safe to infer that they do not affect nerve conduction. Recent work (see Kuffler, 1967) suggests that they could exert considerable influence on synaptic transmission but the definitive experiments remain to be done. The oligodendrocytes, however, are known to produce the myelin sheaths which invest many central axons and function to raise their conduction velocity. It is this fatty sheath which distinguishes the white matter from the non-myelinated cell bodies and axons which compose the grey matter. Peripheral nerve fibres are also overlaid with glial cells, called Schwann cells,

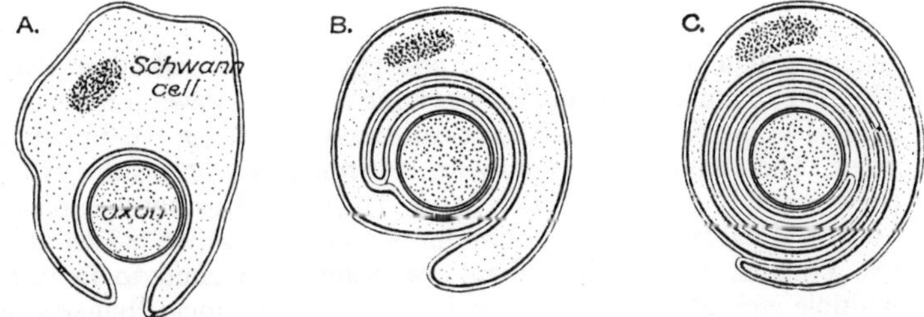

FIG. 4. A diagram of a nerve fibre and its Schwann cell, showing stages in the formation of the myelin sheath.

and again these frequently spiral round the axons, producing a myelin sheath.

Recording Nervous Activity

The signals carried about the nervous system take the form of discrete electrical disturbances which propagate along the axons without decrement. The magnitude of these signals, like the cables

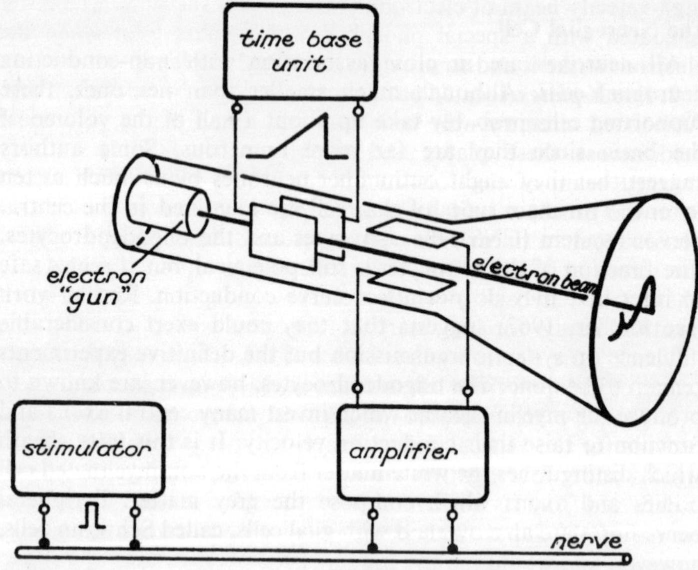

FIG. 5. The cathode ray oscilloscope (CRO) is the conventional instrument used to display nervous activity. The vacuum tube of the CRO contains an electron "gun" which directs a focussed beam of electrons at a fluorescent screen, and two pairs of deflection plates. The timebase unit generates a "sawtooth" voltage waveform which is applied to the X-plates and directs the electron beam in the horizontal plane. The stimulator is simply an electronic pulse generator which is being used here to activate a nerve. The nervous response is picked up with suitable recording electrodes, amplified and then passed on to the Y-plates. Often, more than one beam is required to facilitate multiple recordings, stimulus monitoring, etc. Additional channels can be provided by inserting a further electron "gun" and deflection plates or—more economically—by splitting the original beam into two halves which share common X-plates but independent Y-plates.

along which they travel, is small, and special equipment is required to record them. Many of the experimental results which will be considered later are presented as a photograph of a trace on the screen of a cathode ray oscilloscope. This instrument provides a convenient visual display of the time course of transient electrical signals and is therefore widely used to display nervous activity. It consists essentially of three parts:

1. *An evacuated tube:* contains an electron gun which directs a high-velocity beam of electrons at the face of the tube. The latter is coated with a special phosphor which emits light when the electrons strike it and so provides the visual display.

2. *Two X-plates:* located one on each side of the beam of electrons. Associated circuitry—the timebase unit—generates an electrical field across these plates and thereby deflects the negatively charged beam of electrons in the horizontal plane. The output from the timebase unit has a sawtooth waveform in which two phases recur: a linear rising phase which sweeps the spot across the screen at a steady velocity, followed by a very rapid decay phase (the "flyback") which returns the spot to its original position ready for the start of the next sweep. During the "flyback", the electron gun is switched off so that only the linear sweep of the spot, from left to right, is visible on the screen.

3. *Two Y-plates:* located above and below the beam, these provide for the vertical deflection of the spot. When the voltage signals under investigation are applied to these plates, the beam is deflected from its horizontal traverse and so traces out the time course of the input. The basic instrument is rather insensitive however, and would require inputs of the order of tens of volts to produce appreciable deflections. For this reason, incoming signals are first amplified before being passed on to the Y-plates.

The Nerve Impulse

The ordinary peripheral nerves familiar to the dissector may contain several hundred individual axons, both motor and sensory. In vertebrates, the largest of these are only 20 microns in diameter, so that the isolation of single fibres for recording purposes necessitates careful dissection under a microscope. Fig. 6 illustrates one such experiment in which electrical activity is recorded from the axon of a muscle stretch receptor. The application of a force to the muscle tendon evokes a train of identical nerve impulses in the axon. Each of these impulses is very brief, the main part of the spike lasting about 1 millisecond. Varying the intensity of the stimulus by altering the force applied to the tendon is without effect on the form of each impulse and merely alters the rate at which they are generated. Once initiated, the nerve impulse is a self-regenerating phenomenon, propagating along the fibre by

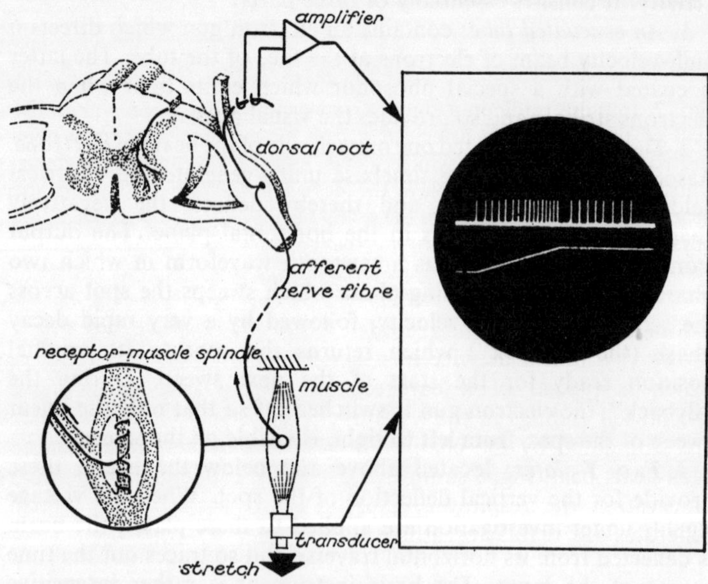

FIG. 6. Recording the activity in a single receptor axon. In this particular preparation, the individual axon is dissected free by successive paring of a filament from the dorsal root and the impulses are led off to an amplifier for display on the upper beam of a CRO. The receptor—a muscle spindle—is activated by a pull on the muscle which is transmitted through a transducer. This device converts the tension changes into equivalent electrical signals which can be monitored on the lower beam of the CRO. Note that the timebase velocity is such that the sweep takes just over half a second. (After Crowe & Matthews, 1964.)

drawing upon the resources of the axon itself. In this respect, the passage of the impulse can be likened to the spread of a flame along a trail of gunpowder, where each grain is ignited by the heat from the one before. The characteristics of the nerve impulse are therefore determined by the properties of the axon and are independent of the means by which they are generated.

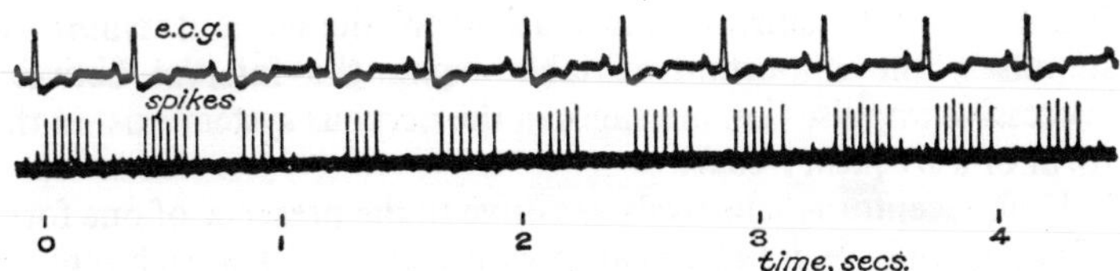

FIG. 7. Impulse traffic in a single axon coming from a receptor in the wall of the pulmonary artery of a dog. The upper trace shows the electrocardiogram (e.c.g.) which signals each contraction of the heart, whilst the lower trace displays the action potentials. Each time the heart ejects blood, the walls of the pulmonary artery are distended and a burst of impulses is initiated at the receptor. (Coleridge & Kidd, 1960.)

Similar signals can be recorded from other nerves and Fig. 7 shows rhythmical activity in a single axon of the Vagus nerve which is typical of a baroreceptor fibre. These axons have specialised endings in the walls of the major blood vessels which are stimulated by the changes in blood pressure consequent to each heart beat. Fig. 8 samples the impulse traffic in a single fibre innervating the respiratory muscles. It is such activity which generates our regular breathing movements.

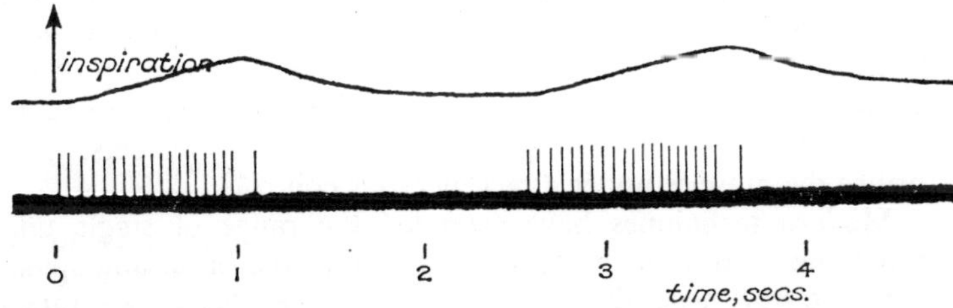

FIG. 8. Impulse activity in one of the motoneurones supplying the diaphragm in a cat. The upper trace shows the pressure in the trachea, a parameter which varies with each breathing movement and provides a convenient monitor of each respiratory cycle. The lower trace shows the phasic impulse activity coincident with, and responsible for, each inspiration. (After Pitts, 1942.)

These experiments reveal that the communication lines in the nervous system deal in one kind of signal only, the nerve impulse, whose repetition rate varies with the intensity of the input. Neurones thus convey information in bursts and trains of impulses, the important variable being the interval between successive impulses i.e. messages in the nervous system exist in the form of a *frequency code*.

Each receptor is selectively sensitive to the presence of one form of energy only (e.g. heat, light, pressure etc.) so that each sensory fibre only carries information relating to some very limited aspect of the environment. On reaching the CNS, the input fibres group together according to the particular modality which they subserve, thereby forming separate pathways for each of the primary sensations. In this way, the CNS separates and classifies incoming signals so that they can be relayed to appropriate processing centres in the brain. Thus, it is possible to consider the "visual pathways" and "visual centres" as discrete areas of the brain concerned chiefly with handling visual information. Similarly, there are "olfactory centres", "auditory centres", "tactile centres" etc. The quality of the sensation aroused by a particular stimulus is therefore determined by the central destination of the activated fibres.

The muscles which move our trunk and limbs work only in response to command signals from the CNS, and the individual muscle fibres have many properties in common with nerve axons including the ability to propagate impulses. The junctions between motor nerve terminals and muscle fibres are very similar in organization to the central inter-neuronal synapses, and function to generate impulses in the muscle. Contraction of the muscle follows in the wake of these impulses, which serve to synchronize the shortening of the contractile elements. This brings the muscles under direct, nervous control.

Modern techniques have extended the range of single unit recordings and even those neurones within the brain and spinal cord are now accessible to study. Central cell bodies are rarely more than a few tens of microns across, and it is necessary to miniaturise the pick-up electrodes if recordings from this central mass are to be restricted to single neurones only. Micropipettes are frequently used for this purpose, being drawn from fine glass tubing to achieve a tip diameter of less than a micron. When filled with a good conducting fluid such as concentrated NaCl or KCl, the tip can be lowered into the brain tissue to record the electrical activity in the vicinity of a single cell body or axon. With sufficient care, these electrodes can even penetrate to the interior of the cell without seriously interfering with its activity. Such recordings have provided considerable information about the functional organization of central synapses.

CHAPTER 2

The Resting Nerve

The ability of the neurone to support impulses rests in part on its ability to establish a high-energy state during periods of inactivity. The propagation of impulses involves the neurone in an expenditure of energy which it meets by drawing upon these reserves. A necessary first step, therefore, in any consideration of nervous activity, is to examine conditions in the quiescent nerve. The small size of mammalian neurones makes them difficult to manipulate and has led many workers to use the larger structures found in invertebrate material. Most of the evidence which will be presented here comes from experiments on the giant axons of the squid. These axons commonly have diameters of half a millimeter or more, and although this is very large, particularly by mammalian standards, they nonetheless seem to function in the same way as most other nerve and muscle fibres.

The Resting Potential

A universal finding in excitable cells is the existence of an electrical potential gradient across the boundary membranes, *the membrane potential*. This steady potential difference between the inside and the outside of the cell can be measured with an oscilloscope and a suitable amplifier. Thus, impaling axons with a micropipette reveals a resting membrane potential which varies slightly in magnitude from one neurone to another but is usually about 60 millivolts (mV), with the inside always *negatively* charged with respect to the outside. Suitable electrical stimulation of the axon will initiate nerve impulses, during which there is a brief reversal of the membrane potential.

Analysis of the axoplasm shows that, like most cells, the neurone contains significantly more potassium ions and organic anions than either the blood or seawater (seawater is the blood-substitute usually employed in experiments). Conversely, the cell contains significantly less sodium ions and chloride ions.

The concentrations given in Table 1 show little variation over long periods of time in quiescent axons and represent the steady-state conditions in the nerve. The maintenance of such an unequal distribution of ions across the membrane might suggest that there

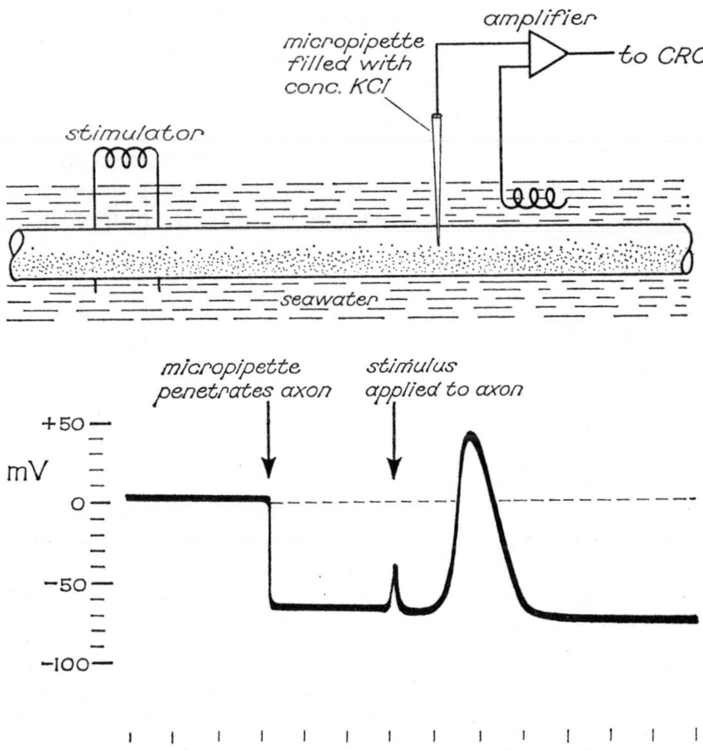

FIG. 9. An intracellular recording from a squid giant axon. As the miniaturized probe (in the form of a micropipette with a tip diameter of less than 1 micron) penetrates the axon membrane, a shift in the baseline of the CRO beam indicates a membrane potential of about – 70mV. Electrical stimulation of the axon generates an action potential, during which the membrane potential is briefly reversed. (After Hodgkin, 1958.)

is only a very restricted exchange between the axoplasm and the external medium but this is only partly true, and underestimates the complexity of the situation. Before examining this statement further, it is necessary to consider some physicochemical aspects which are important in the system.

TABLE 1

Concentrations of the chief ions in the squid axon.
(After Hodgkin, 1964)

Substance	Concentration (mmole/kg H_2O)		
	Axoplasm	Blood	Seawater
K	400	20	10
Na	50	440	460
Cl	120	560	540
Organic anions —mainly isethionate	360	—	—

The Movement of Ions through Solutions and Membranes

All molecules are in a continual state of thermal agitation. Molecules in solution are relatively free to move about so that these random vibrations tend to disperse them evenly throughout the medium. If there is a non-uniform distribution of molecules in a solution, then these kinetic or diffusional forces cause a net migration down the concentration gradients. Although molecules in fact move in all directions through the medium, our main concern is only with the net flux i.e. the extent to which the rate of the forward migration exceeds the reverse movement and so produces a net transfer. The rate at which this net migration proceeds will of course depend upon the concentration differences within the solution.

Since ions are charged, they are also influenced by electrical gradients. The ions in the neurone are subject to both electrical and chemical (concentration) gradients and the magnitude and direction of the net transfer of a given ionic species must reflect the resultant of these two vectors.

Different ions have different rates of migration, even when subjected to the same driving force. Thus, Na ions migrate just over 5 microns every second in a field of 1 volt per centimeter, whilst in similar circumstances, K ions and Cl ions travel almost 8 microns. This may seem puzzling at first, since the Na ion is the smallest of the three and might, therefore, have been expected to encounter less resistance to movement than the larger K and

Cl ions. However, the ease with which ions move through aqueous solution—their *mobility*—depends to a large extent upon their degree of hydration i.e. the size of the "shell" of water molecules which they transport with them. The small Na ion is more hydrated, and therefore has a greater "functional" size, than the K ion and Cl ion, thus accounting for their apparently anomalous mobilities.

From this, it should be evident that the net flux, or rate of migration, of a given ionic species in solution is a function of its mobility and the electrochemical gradient which it experiences. These factors must also be considered in the movement of ions across membranes, though a slightly different approach is used. Here, it is more usual to refer to the *permeability* of the membrane to a particular ion than to the mobility of that ion in the mem

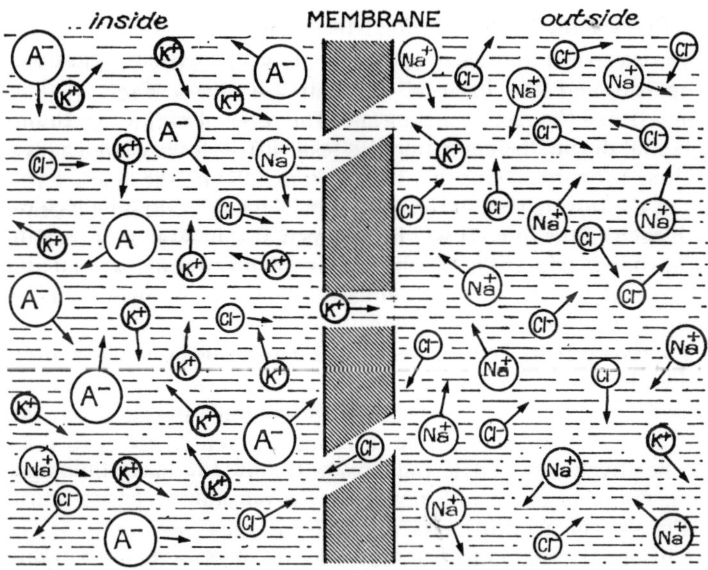

FIG. 10. An impression of the resting nerve membrane, showing pores large enough to allow K and Cl ions to penetrate fairly readily whilst giving only restricted passage to Na ions and none at all to A ions. Although the notion of "pores" is an oversimplification, such a model can often provide a useful conceptual basis when considering passive interchanges between the two ionic populations.

brane. Both of these terms refer to the ease with which a given ion will pass through the membrane, and will therefore depend upon the relative dimensions of the hydrated ion and the pores in the membrane through which it is obliged to travel. The differences between the functional sizes of the various ions enables membranes to discriminate between them. Thus, a membrane with a suitably sized pore could permit free passage of the smaller hydrated K ions and Cl ions, whilst providing a virtually impenetrable barrier to the larger Na ions. When describing the permeability of the membrane therefore, it is necessary to specify the ions involved e.g. in the above case, the membrane has a high permeability to K ions and Cl ions and a low permeability to Na ions. The membrane of the neurone, however, does not always conform to the simple, sieve-like structure assumed above and other factors must be invoked to explain its permeability function.

The Permeability of the Resting Membrane

The electrical and chemical gradients which exist between the axoplasm and the external medium are due entirely to the properties of the resting membrane. The reversal of the membrane potential during the nerve impulse results from a transient change in these properties. Our first task is to investigate the characteristics of the resting membrane and, in particular, to see how it deals with each of the ions. It will be assumed at this stage that there is independent migration of ions across the membrane, so that the passage of the ion in question can be assumed to proceed as if there were no other ions present.

Potassium Ions. The K ions exist in much higher concentration inside the neurone than outside, hence there is a net tendency for them to leak out along this concentration gradient. However, the electrical gradient due to the membrane potential tends to hold the positively charged K ions inside the axon—the inside being some 60mV negative with respect to the outside.

Clearly, the net diffusional and electrostatic forces on the K ion are in opposition, and since they are expressed in different units, it is not immediately obvious which one is going to have the greater influence. In order to determine the net driving force on the K ion, the concentration gradient is converted into electrical terms i.e. it is expressed as an equivalent electrical gradient. Only then can we assess the relative magnitudes of the two influences. This can be done simply, though rather indirectly, by means of a conversion factor in the form of *the Nernst Equation,* which is stated in full below:

$$\text{electrical gradient (in volts)} = \frac{RT}{FZ} \cdot \log_e \frac{[\text{ion}]_o}{[\text{ion}]_i}.$$

where

R = universal gas constant (8·31 joules/mol/°absolute)
F = the faraday (96,500 coulombs/mol)
T = temperature in °absolute
Z = valence of the ion
$[\text{ion}]_o$ = concentration of the ion outside the cell
$[\text{ion}]_i$ = concentration of the ion inside the cell

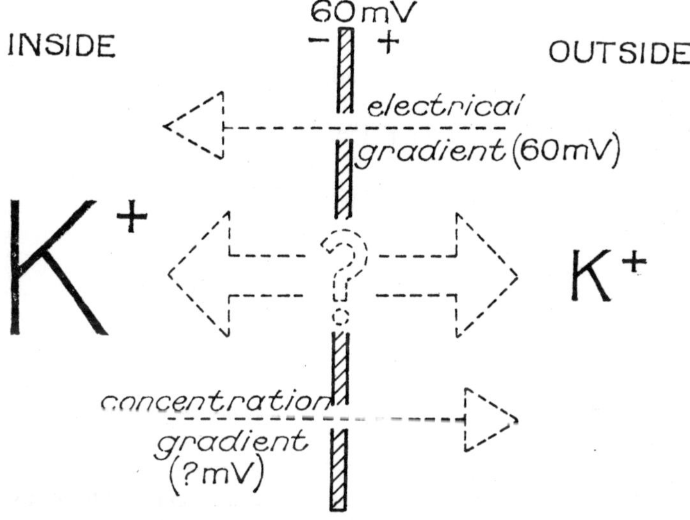

FIG. 11. The forces on the K ions in the resting squid axon. The net driving force, or electrochemical gradient, experienced by the K ions is determined by two factors: the *electrical* gradient due to the membrane potential and the *chemical* gradient due to concentration differences across the membrane. Clearly, in the case of the K ions in the squid axon, these two gradients are in opposition and in order to resolve the net effect, both gradients must be expressed in the same units. It is usual to employ the electrical units for both gradients, hence the immediate problem is to convert the concentration gradient into an equivalent electrical one.

The equation can be simplified by substituting for the various constants. Thus, in the case of a monovalent ion such as the K ion, assuming a temperature of 18°C:

$$\text{electrical gradient (in volts)} = \frac{8{\cdot}31\,.\,291}{96{,}500\,.\,1}\,.\,\log_e \frac{[\mathrm{K}]_o}{[\mathrm{K}]_i}$$

Converting to logarithms to the base ten and multiplying by 1000 to give the result in millivolts (mV):

$$\text{electrical gradient (in mV)} = \frac{8{\cdot}31\,.\,291\,.\,2{\cdot}303\,.\,1000}{96{,}500\,.\,1}\,.\,\log_{10} \frac{[\mathrm{K}]_o}{[\mathrm{K}]_i}$$

$$= 58\,.\,\log_{10} \frac{[\mathrm{K}]_o}{[\mathrm{K}]_i} \quad \text{(approx.)}$$

This simplified form of the Nernst Equation provides the magnitude of the electrical gradient which would have to be applied to exactly balance the forces due to the concentration gradient. In the case of the K ions in the squid axon:

$$[\mathrm{K}]_o = 20 \text{ mmole/kg } H_2O$$
$$[\mathrm{K}]_i = 400 \text{ mmole/kg } H_2O$$

whence

$$\text{electrical gradient (in mV)} = 58\,.\,\log_{10} \frac{20}{400}$$
$$= 58\,.\,\log_{10} 0{\cdot}05$$
$$= 58\,.\,\bar{2}{\cdot}6990$$
$$= (58\,.\,-2)+(58\,.\,0{\cdot}6990)$$
$$= -75 \text{ mV} \quad \text{(approx.)}.$$

This indicates, that if the membrane potential was changed to −75 mV, i.e. the inside was made 75 mV *negative* with respect to the outside, then the resulting electrostatic forces on the K ions would exactly balance the diffusional forces arising from the concentration gradient (see Fig 12).

Under these circumstances, even if the membrane was assumed to be permeable to K ions, there would be no net flux since the tendency for the K ions to leak out on the concentration gradient has been exactly offset by the electrical gradient (membrane potential) viz. the electrochemical gradient is zero. The K ions would therefore be in equilibrium, with influx = efflux. For this reason, the potential difference calculated from the Nernst Equation is termed *the equilibrium potential for the* K *ion.*

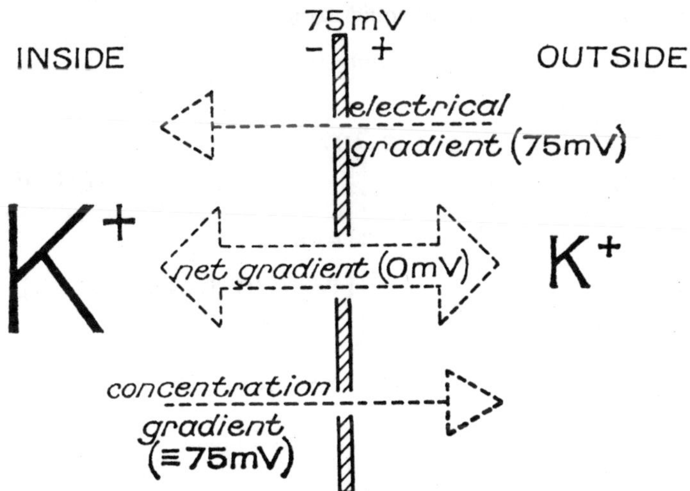

FIG. 12. The equilibrium condition, when the electrochemical gradient for the K ion is zero. The Nernst equation has been used to express the concentration gradient as an equivalent electrical gradient (approximately 75mV). If now the membrane potential is adjusted to − 75mV (i.e. the inside negative with respect to the outside) the tendency for the K ions to move in under this electrical gradient exactly counterbalances the tendency to move out on the concentration gradient, whence efflux will be equal to influx.

Thus, in the squid axon, the K concentration gradient exerts net *diffusional* forces which are equivalent to the *electrostatic* forces which would be produced by an electrical gradient of 75 mV. With a normal resting membrane potential of −60 mV, the concentration gradient predominates by the equivalent of some 15 mV i.e. the K ions will experience a net driving force which tends to move them out of the cell:

net driving force on K ions (mV)

$$= \begin{array}{c}\text{electrical gradient}\\ \text{on K ions}\end{array} - \begin{array}{c}\text{concentration gradient}\\ \text{for K ions}\end{array}$$

$$= \begin{array}{c}\text{membrane potential}\\ (E_m)\end{array} - \begin{array}{c}\text{equilibrium potential}\\ \text{for K ions } (E_K)\end{array}$$

$$= E_m - E_K.$$

Therefore, in the quiescent squid axon,

$$\text{net driving force on K ions (mV)} = (-60)-(-75) = +15 \text{ mV}.$$

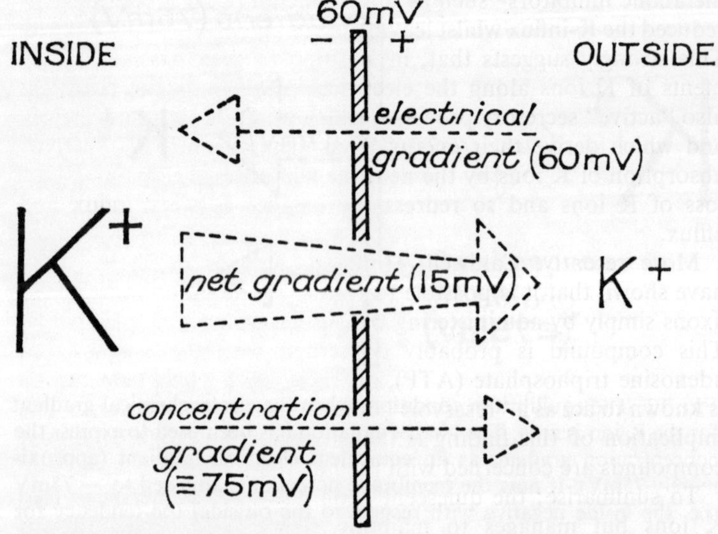

FIG. 13. In the resting squid axon, there is a net gradient which tends to move K ions out of the axon.

Using radioactive isotopes of potassium (K^{42}), Keynes (1951a & b.) and Keynes & Lewis (1951a & b.) showed that the K ions in crab and cuttlefish axons are in continuous flux across the quiescent membrane. Shanes & Berman (1955) subsequently applied these tracer techniques to squid axons with similar results. These findings show that nerve membranes are indeed permeable to K ions and therefore present us with some difficulties since our calculations indicate that under these circumstances there should be a steady net loss of K ions. In order to explain how the resting concentration gradients are maintained, we must postulate some system which can make up for this passive K-loss by pumping K ions back into the axon. Such a process would require a source of energy since it would be transporting K ions against the prevailing electrochemical gradient and must, therefore, perform work.

In designing experiments to test this hypothesis, a reasonable first assumption is that such a system would derive its energy ultimately from the metabolic oxidation of foodstuffs. In further tracer experiments, Hodgkin & Keynes (1955a) found that metabolic inhibitors* such as dinitrophenol (DNP), considerably reduced the K-influx whilst leaving the K-efflux almost unchanged. This strongly suggests that, in addition to the "passive" movements of K ions along the electrochemical gradients, there are also "active" secretory processes which pump K ions into the cell and which derive their energy from metabolism. This "active" absorption of K ions by the neurone will offset the "passive" net loss of K ions and so redress the balance between influx and efflux.

More recently, Caldwell, Hodgkin, Keynes & Shaw (1960) have shown that it is possible to restore the K-influx in poisoned axons simply by administering the substance arginine phosphate. This compound is probably concerned with the synthesis of adenosine triphosphate (ATP), an energy-rich phosphate, which is known to act as a "reservoir" of energy in many other cells. The implication of this finding is that arginine phosphate or similar compounds are concerned with fuelling the K-pump.

To summarise: the quiescent axon has a net tendency to lose K ions but manages to maintain steady-state concentrations through an "active" transport mechanism which moves K ions into the axon.

In poisoned axons, the movements of the K ions are determined entirely by the "passive" electrical and chemical gradients, and the expected flux ratio (efflux : influx) is about 2·5 : 1. However, the flux ratios found in poisoned cuttlefish axons were much greater than this—about 10 : 1. It seems that this exaggerated flux ratio is due to interaction between the incoming and outgoing currents in the K channels (Hodgkin & Keynes, 1955b.) This refutes one of our earlier assumptions—that there is independent migration of ions across the membrane—at least so far as the K ions in cuttlefish axons are concerned, and suggests that the membrane has a more complex structure than was assumed above.

*Amongst other things, these substances block the production of energy-rich phosphate compounds such as ATP. Thus, any process which requires energy and is normally "fuelled" by these phosphate compounds, will gradually fail after the administration of inhibitors.

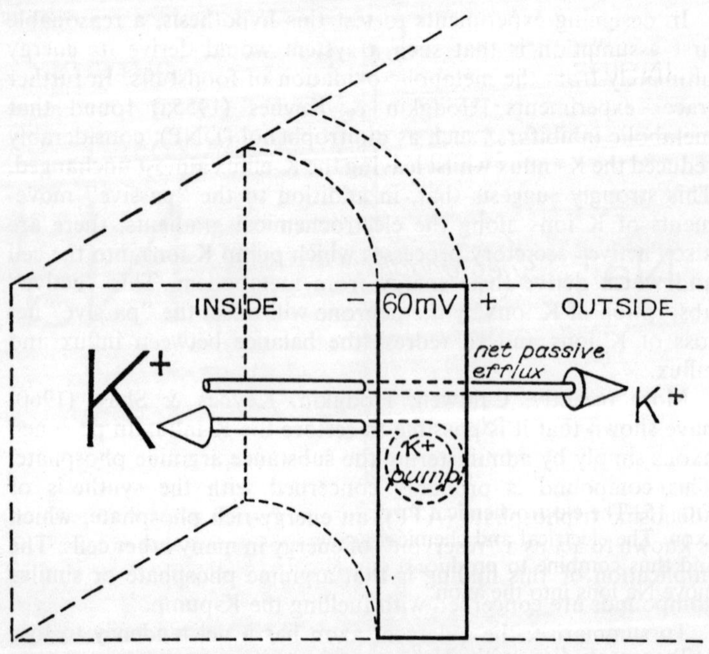

FIG. 14. A summary of the K-fluxes in the resting squid axon. The net (passive) K-loss is offset by active K-uptake.

Sodium Ions. It is not necessary to perform any calculations to see that there is a considerable electrochemical gradient tending to drive Na ions into the axon. Both the electrical and the net chemical gradients promote an uptake of Na ions by the neurone. Substitution in the Nernst Equation shows that the equilibrium potential for the Na ion in the squid axon is +50 mV i.e. the inside would need to be charged 50 mV *positive* with respect to the outside to hold the Na ions in equilibrium. Thus, the concentration gradient is equivalent to an electrical gradient of 50 mV and, taken together with the normal resting membrane potential, provides a total net driving force on the Na ion of 110 mV:

$$\begin{aligned}\text{net driving force on Na ion} &= E_m - E_{Na}\\ &= (-60)-(+50)\\ &= -110 \text{ mV.}\end{aligned}$$

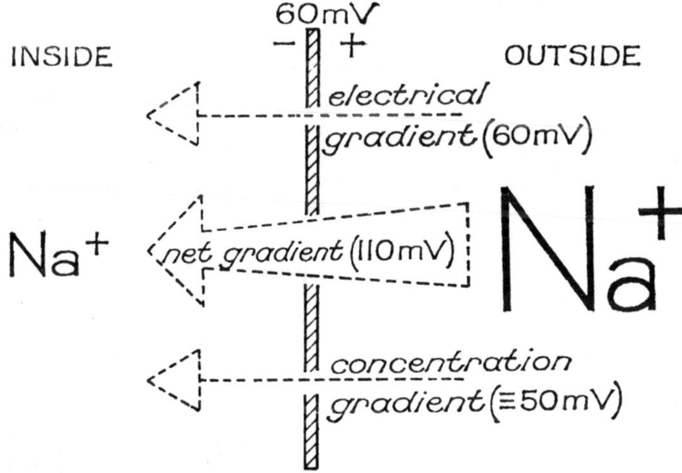

FIG. 15. The electrochemical forces on the Na ion in the resting squid axon. The electrical and chemical gradients are both directed inwards and thus combine to produce a considerable driving force tending to move Na ions into the axon.

Tracer studies with Na^{24} reveal that the membrane of the quiescent squid axon is slightly permeable to Na ions and permits an exchange between the axoplasm and the external solution (Shanes & Berman, 1955). However, it is apparent from our calculations that the net "passive" forces would lead to a migration of Na ions into the axon unless countered by an "active" Na-extrusion. Evidence for the up-hill movement of Na ions from the axoplasm into the bathing solution was provided by Hodgkin & Keynes (1955a), who found that DNP selectively suppressed the Na-efflux whilst sparing the Na-influx. Furthermore, the addition of ATP to poisoned axons restored the Na-efflux, at least in part (Caldwell *et al.*, 1960). Thus, again we have a situation in which steady-state concentrations are maintained by an "active" pumping mechanism which counterbalances "passive" leakage currents.

There is some evidence which suggests that the "active" transport mechanisms carrying Na and K ions across the membrane are loosely coupled together as a single Na-K exchange pump. The "active" Na-efflux is reduced to about one third of its

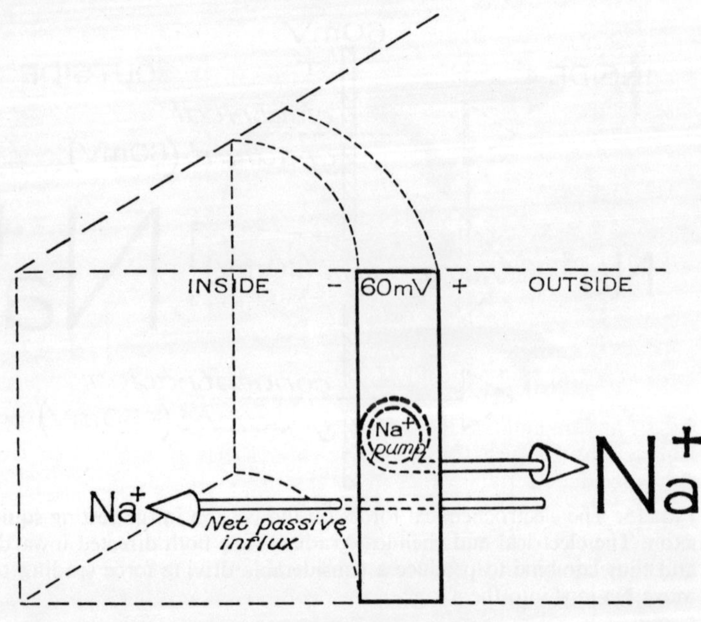

FIG. 16. A summary of the Na-fluxes in the resting squid axon. The net (passive) Na-gain is offset by active Na-extrusion.

normal level when K ions are removed from the external solution, whilst raising $[K]_o$ produced an increase in the Na-efflux (Hodgkin & Keynes, 1955a). It is not difficult to appreciate how an alteration in the number of K ions outside the axon and hence available for "active" transport into the axon, can alter the K pumping rate. However, the finding that such adjustments in the K-pumping rate are accompanied by similar fluctuations in the active transport of Na ions suggests that the two "active" processes are linked in some way (see Fig. 17).

The reduction in Na-efflux which follows the withdrawal of K ions from the external solution is about equal to the reduction in K-influx produced by DNP i.e. arresting the K-pump reduces the Na-pumping rate by an amount just equal to the normal K-pumping rate. Presumeably, therefore, the coupled Na-K transport mechanism is a one-for-one exchange with each K ion being exchanged for a Na ion. However, this exchange pump does

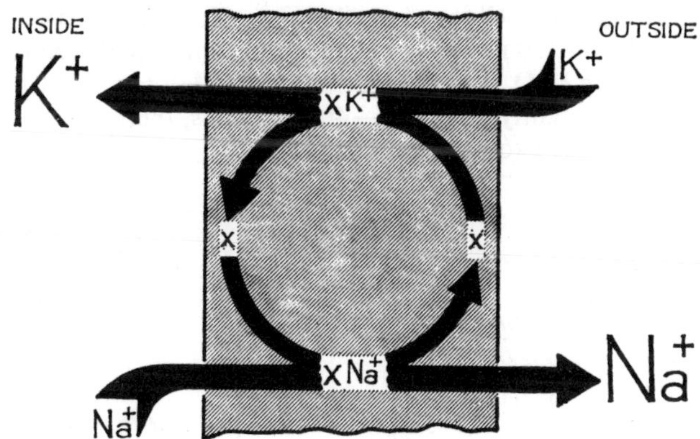

FIG. 17. Coupling of the active Na and K transport mechanisms. Interactions between the active Na- and K-fluxes suggest that they probably share certain carrier molecules (X).

not account for all of the Na ions which are "actively" moved out of the neurone since the reduction in Na-efflux following removal of external K ions is less than that produced by DNP.

Throughout this discussion, we have assumed that the pump mechanisms reside within the membrane. This is supported by many findings, but in particular, the experiments of Baker, Hodgkin & Shaw (1962) leave little alternative. These workers showed that the axoplasm in the squid axon could be almost completely replaced by isotonic solutions of various K salts with little effect on either the membrane potential or the excitability of the neurone. On the other hand, even slight damage to the membrane caused a rapid deterioration.

Chloride Ions. The chloride fluxes in the squid axon seem to differ from those in other nerve and muscle fibres which have been researched, but the functional significance of this is not clear at the present time. There is considerable evidence showing that the membrane of the frog skeletal muscle fibre is about twice as permeable to Cl ions as it is to K ions (Hodgkin & Horowicz, 1959; Hutter & Noble, 1960) and that the Cl ions are equilibrated i.e. $E_{Cl} = E_m$ (Adrian, 1960, 1961). Thus, no "active" transport mechanisms are involved in this case. However, Keynes (1963) found that the Cl ion concentration in the squid axon is much too high for these ions to be equilibrated, suggesting that there must be up-hill transport of Cl ions into the axon. Keynes estimated $[\text{Cl}]_i$ to be about 120 mmole/kg.H_2O, and with $[\text{Cl}]_o$ equal to 560 mmole/kg.H_2O, the equilibrium potential for the Cl ions works out at slightly less than −40 mV. Thus, there will be a net tendency for the axon to lose Cl ions:

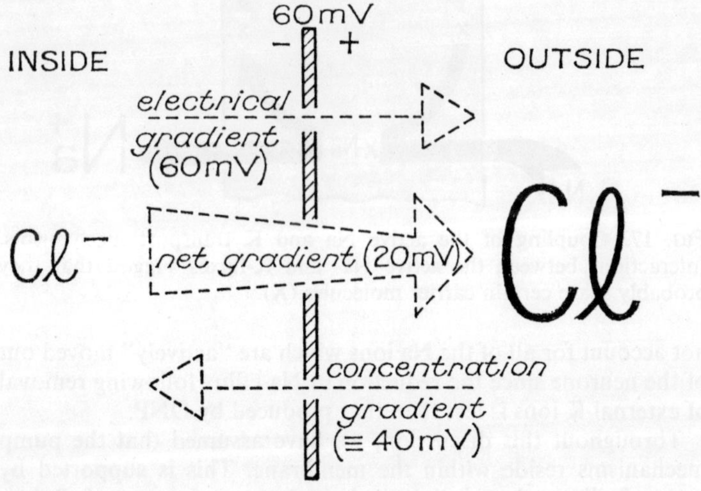

FIG. 18. The electrochemical forces on the Cl ion in the resting squid axon, showing the net tendency for Cl ions to leak out of the axon.

Keynes deduced the Cl-permeability of the squid axon membrane to be less than a fifth of the K-permeability and found that the Cl-influx was halved by DNP. Once again, it seems that the steady-state is maintained by "active" transport processes in the membrane.

The only other ions which are of relevance to us here are the large organic anions in the axoplasm, the chief of which in squid axon, is isethionic acid (Koechlin, 1955). These ions appear to be much too large to penetrate the membrane and remain trapped inside the cell.

The Origin of the Resting Membrane Potential

So far, we have only considered the steady-state condition in the neurone in which a dynamic equilibrium maintains fairly constant

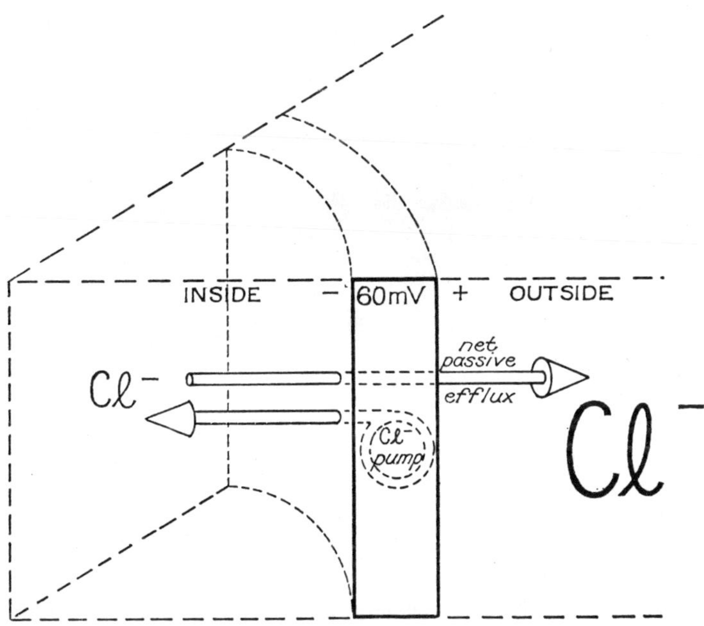

FIG. 19. A summary of the Cl-fluxes in the resting squid axon. The net (passive) Cl-loss is offset by active Cl-uptake.

electrical and chemical gradients across the membrane. Our next task is to find out how these gradients arise.

The chemical gradients originate from the activity of the Na-K exchange pump. (The contribution of the Cl-pump is only of minor significance and, initially at least, can be ignored.) In order to elucidate the mechanisms involved, let us consider a simplified, hypothetical situation in which initially there are no gradients across the membrane. Thus, suppose that identical solutions containing a mixture of KCl and NaCl in equal proportions, are placed on each side of the membrane. When the coupled Na-K pump comes into operation, concentration gradients will be established for these ions, but if for the present we assume the pump to be electrically neutral—merely exchanging cation for cation—then no electrical gradient will result directly from this.

However, the ionic gradients generated by the "active" trans-

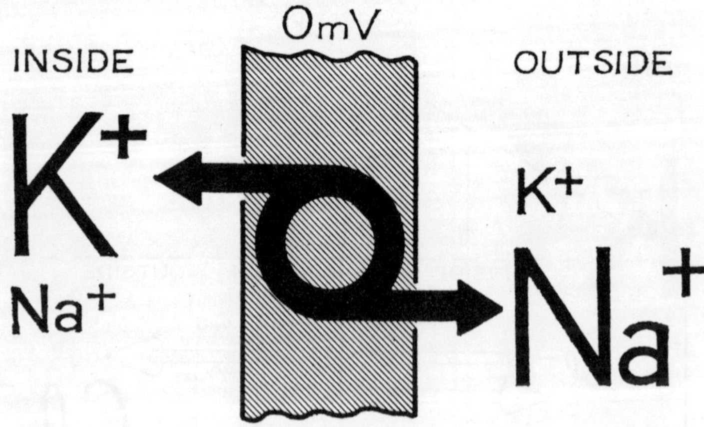

FIG. 20. The Na and K concentration gradients are established by the exchange pump which derives the necessary energy from the metabolic breakdown of foodstuffs.

port now provide the necessary driving forces for a "passive" back-diffusion of Na and K ions i.e. there will be a "passive" K-loss and Na-gain. Having assumed that the pump is a one-for-one exchange of Na ions for K ions, it follows that the concentration gradients generated by the pump will be the same for the two ions and hence they will experience the same driving forces. Nonetheless, the "passive" K-loss proceeds at a much greater rate than the "passive" Na-gain because the membrane is far more permeable to the K ions. Hodgkin & Katz (1949) estimate that the resting membrane is at least 25 times more permeable to K ions than to Na ions. There is thus a net loss of cations (K ions) from the cell which charges up the membrane so that the inside is negative with respect to the outside.

The magnitude of this membrane potential will depend upon (*a*) the pumping rate, and (*b*) the disparity between the K- and Na-permeabilities of the membrane (P_K and P_{Na}). The greater the ratio $P_K : P_{Na}$, then the greater the inequality in the back-diffusion of these ions and, therefore, the greater the separation of charge. (To a first approximation, the resting membrane can be regarded as impermeable to all ions except potassium. The magnitude of the resting potential is therefore determined

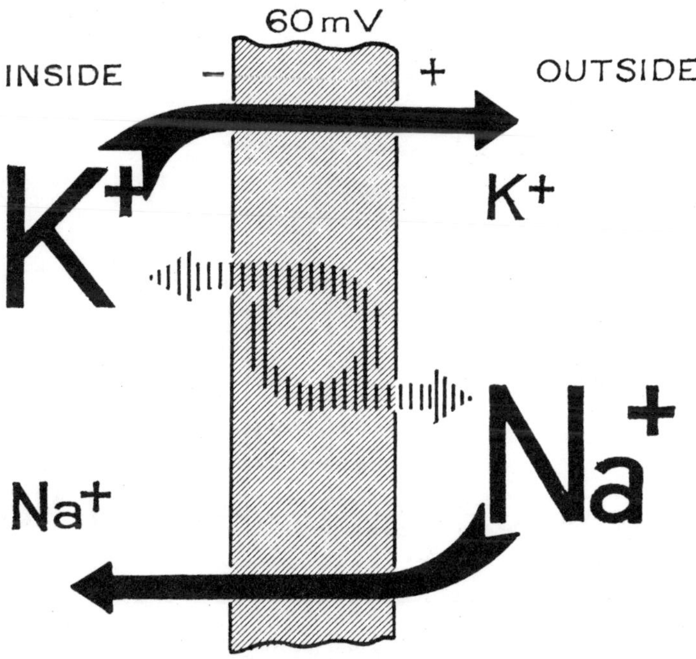

FIG. 21. The concentration gradients established by the exchange pump promote the diffusion of Na and K ions back across the membrane. Since the membrane is much more permeable to the K ions, back-diffusion of the K ion proceeds more rapidly than back-diffusion of the Na ion, resulting in a net loss of cations and the development of a potential difference across the membrane such that the inside is negative with respect to the outside.

largely by the potassium concentration gradient.) The developing electrical gradient, however, operates against the "passive" K-loss whilst encouraging the "passive" Na-gain. As the membrane potential rises therefore, it brings about a progressive decrease in the disparity between the Na and K fluxes. Eventually, an equilibrium is established and for each ion, the efflux balances the influx.

Any slight deviation of the membrane potential away from this resting level immediately uncovers driving forces which promote ionic currents across the membrane to restore the equilibrium,

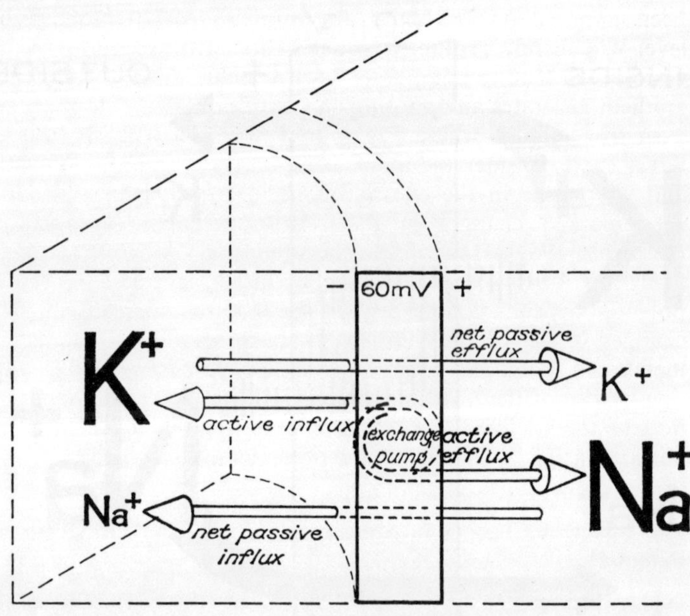

FIG. 22. A summary of the active and passive movements of Na and K in the resting squid axon.

e.g. a rise in membrane potential (which represents a rise in the electrical gradient on each ion) disturbs the balance of forces on the Na and K ions in favour of an increased cation influx which then operates to re-establish the resting potential. Thus, the resting nerve is in a state of stable equilibrium.

Although the membrane of the squid axon is relatively impermeable to Cl ions ($P_K : P_{Cl} = 5{\cdot}6 : 1$ approx.) it is nonetheless clear that some of these ions will penetrate the membrane. During the genesis of the membrane potential, when the net cation loss is charging up the membrane, Cl ions will be moving out of the axon along the electrical gradient. This means that some of the K ions lost from the axon will be accompanied by Cl ions, thereby reducing the effective charge separation. The Cl ions thus tend to prevent the membrane potential reaching the equilibrium level referred to above. However, this setback in the development of the potential is less significant than might have been supposed. As seen above, any failure to reach the equilibrium level will merely prolong the net cation loss. In addition, the Cl ions will tend to equilibrate as their efflux down the electrical gradient generates an opposing concentration gradient.

In frog muscle, where P_{Cl} is high ($P_{Cl} : P_K = 2 : 1$), the Cl-fluxes exert considerable influence upon the membrane potential and alterations in the chloride concentration gradient produce very marked changes in the resting potential (Hodgkin & Horowicz, 1959). However, in the squid axon, where P_{Cl} is relatively low, Cl ions are only of minor importance and the resting potential depends very largely on the K ion gradient. Even large changes in the Cl ion gradient produce very small changes in membrane potential (Baker, Hodgkin & Shaw, 1962). The significance of the Cl-pump which raises the internal concentration of the Cl ions is not known and seems to have little importance as far as the membrane potential is concerned.

The Effect of Changes in Membrane Permeability on Membrane Potential

It will be seen in subsequent chapters that the excitability of the neurone results largely from its capacity to undergo transient changes in permeability. The "passive" ionic currents which are allowed to flow as a result of these changes produce marked alterations in the transmembrane potential. It will be remembered from the previous section that the membrane potential is a function of the ratio $P_K : P_{Na}$ and that in the resting nerve this ratio is about 25 : 1. Under these conditions, there is an unbalanced loss of cations (K ions) which leaves the inside of the axon negatively charged with respect to the outside. If this situation is reversed and the membrane favours the passage of the Na ions whilst discriminating against the K ions, then the "passive" Na-gain will now exceed the "passive" K-loss and the membrane potential will be reversed. Such permeability changes form the basis for the brief reversal in membrane potential during the nerve impulse.

The normal excursions of the membrane potential rarely exceed 100 mV or so and the number of ions involved in the "passive" ionic currents which produce them represents only a minute fraction of the total number available. The full significance of this point will emerge more strongly from a few simple calculations. Let us start with a rough estimate of how many Na ions or K ions must cross the membrane in order to change the potential by 100 mV:

The membrane investing the neurone can be regarded as the dielectric which separates the two conductors in a capacitance:

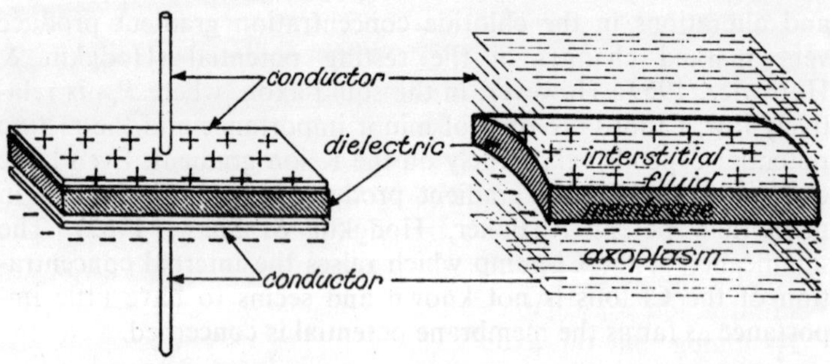

FIG. 23. Changes in membrane potential result from some rearrangement of the charge distribution across the membrane. The numbers of ions (charges) involved in these adjustments naturally depends upon the magnitude of the potential changes and, in addition, upon a property of the membrane known as its capacitance. The capacity of the nerve membrane is a measure of its ability to separate unlike charges and depends upon its insulating properties, thickness and cross-sectional area. The lipoprotein membrane constitutes an insulating barrier (dielectric) between two conducting media and in holding unlike charges apart resembles a simple parallel plate capacitor. (For the moment, we can ignore the "leakage" channels in the membrane.)

The *capacity* of the membrane (in Farads) is a measure of the amount of charge that it will hold (in Coulombs) when a potential difference of 1 Volt exists across it:

$$\text{capacity (farads)} = \frac{\text{quantity of charge (coulombs)}}{\text{potential difference (volts)}}.$$

Experiment shows that the capacity of the squid axon membrane is about 1 microfarad per sq. cm., so that the quantity of charge required to generate a potential difference of 100 mV can now be readily calculated:

$$\begin{aligned}\text{quantity of charge} &= (\text{capacity}).(\text{potential difference}) \\ &= (1.10^{-6}).(100.10^{-3}) \\ &= 10^{-7}\text{coulombs.}\end{aligned}$$

But

$$1 \text{ g. mole} = 96{,}500 \text{ coulombs} = 10^5 \text{ coulombs (approx.).}$$

Whence

$$\begin{aligned}\text{quantity of charge} &= \frac{10^{-7}}{10^5}\text{ g. mole} = 10^{-12}\text{ g. mole} \\ &= 1 \text{ picomole.}\end{aligned}$$

Thus, it only requires the transfer of 1 picomole of Na or K ions across each sq. cm. of the membrane to produce a change in the membrane potential of 100 mV. This is clearly a very small quantity of charge but it now remains to be seen how much Na and K ion is available in the axoplasm:

Assuming that the axon has a diameter of 500 microns, the volume enclosed by 1 sq. cm. of membrane is about 1/80 ml:

$$\text{area of membrane} = 2\pi RL = A.$$

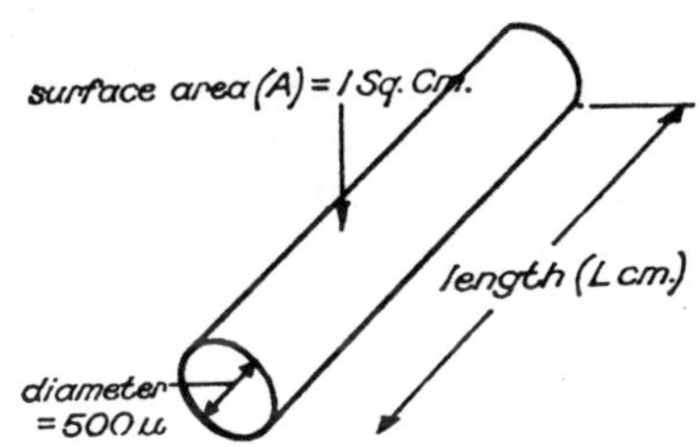

FIG. 24. A section of squid axon.

Whence

$$L = \frac{A}{2\pi R}$$

However

$$\text{volume of the axoplasm} = \pi R^2 L.$$

Substituting for L:

$$\begin{aligned}\text{volume} &= \frac{\pi R^2 A}{2\pi R} \\ &= \frac{RA}{2} \\ &= \frac{0{\cdot}025.1}{2} \\ &= 0{\cdot}0125 \text{ ml.}\end{aligned}$$

However

$$[Na]_i = 50 \text{ mmole/litre} = 5.10^{-5} \text{ mole/ml.}$$

Thus, the quantity of Na ions in the section of axon

$$= 5.10^{-5}.0{\cdot}0125 \text{ mole}$$
$$= 6{\cdot}25.10^{-7} \text{ mole}$$
$$= 625{,}000 \text{ picomoles.}$$

Clearly, an influx of 1 picomole of Na ions would change the membrane potential by 100 mV and would raise $[Na]_i$ by a factor of less than one part in 600,000. Since the K-content of the axoplasm is some 8 times greater than the Na-content, a similar change in membrane potential could result from a K-efflux which would only reduce $[K]_i$ by one part in 5 million!

It will be apparent from this that the axoplasm—and also, in fact, the interstitial fluid bathing the axon—can be regarded as a huge reservoir of ions. The transient excursions in membrane potential which represent activity in the neurone and are generated by "passive" ionic currents, will be accomplished with little immediate effect on the concentration gradients. In addition, since so few ions are involved, these potential changes can be accomplished very quickly—in one or two milliseconds. By contrast the time course of any concentration changes extends over several hours and, in the long term, ionic balance is maintained by the exchange pump. The existence of large reservoirs of ions ensures that the sudden demands for more ions during periods of intense activity can be met. In this respect, it is interesting to note that axons which have been poisoned with metabolic inhibitors, inactivating the exchange pump, can conduct many thousands of impulses before the ionic gradients eventually run down (Hodgkin, 1964).

To summarise: The concentration gradients across the membrane are established by an exchange pump which selectively extrudes Na ions and absorbs K ions. The membrane potential is generated by "passive" Na and K-fluxes along these chemical gradients: K ions tend to leak out of the neurone whilst the Na ions have a strong tendency to move in. The membrane is able to discriminate between these two ions, thereby exerting control over their individual (passive) movements across the membrane. Transient alterations in the permeability of the membrane can thus favour either an efflux or an influx of cations, so that membrane potential is a function of the ratio $P_K : P_{Na}$. When this ratio is high, as it is in the resting neurone, the inside of the membrane is negatively charged due to the net loss of cations. Activation of the membrane reduces the ratio, causing a net cation gain and a reversal of the membrane potential. With large reserves of Na and K ions in the axoplasm and surrounding medium, such movements of charge need only involve a minute proportion of the total number available in order to produce considerable changes in the membrane potential.

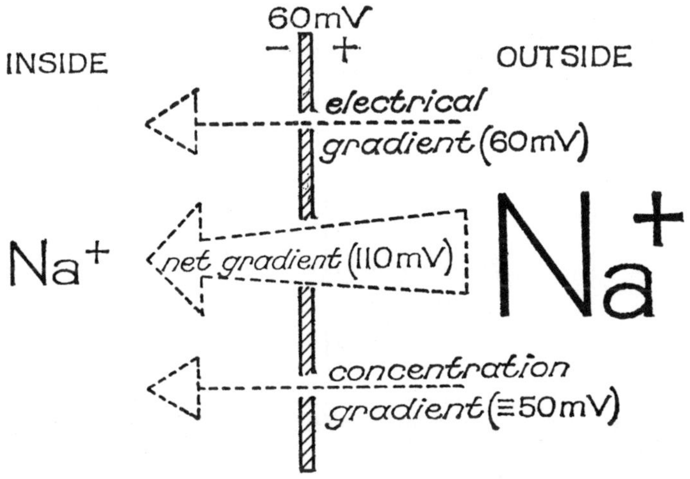

FIG. 25. There is a strong tendency for Na ions to enter the resting nerve and any increase in the permeability of the membrane to this ion will result in a rapid Na-influx.

In certain circumstances, it is relatively easy to make accurate predictions concerning the changes in membrane potential which would follow specific changes in membrane permeability, and it is profitable to look a little further into this aspect.

Suppose that the membrane of the resting squid axon was suddenly rendered very permeable to one particular ion, say the Na ion. Clearly, Na ions would rapidly enter the nerve as a result (see Fig. 25). This influx of cations would reduce the membrane potential and, in so doing, reduce the driving force on which it depends for its existence. As the influx continues therefore, the inside of the axon will become progressively more positive and generate an electrical gradient which will tend to curtail further Na-influx. Eventually, the electrical gradient—membrane potential—will reach a sufficiently positive value to exactly balance the concentration gradient which is tending to drive the Na ions into the axon. The nerve will thus reach a new equilibrium condition. As a result of the Na-influx, the Na concentration gradient will also have fallen but, as pointed out above, only a few of the available ions are involved and the change can be neglected. Thus, the Na concentration gradient can be assumed to remain at its original resting value throughout the exchange and only the membrane potential is involved in these readjustments. It follows therefore, that equilibrium will be established when the electrical gradient (membrane potential)

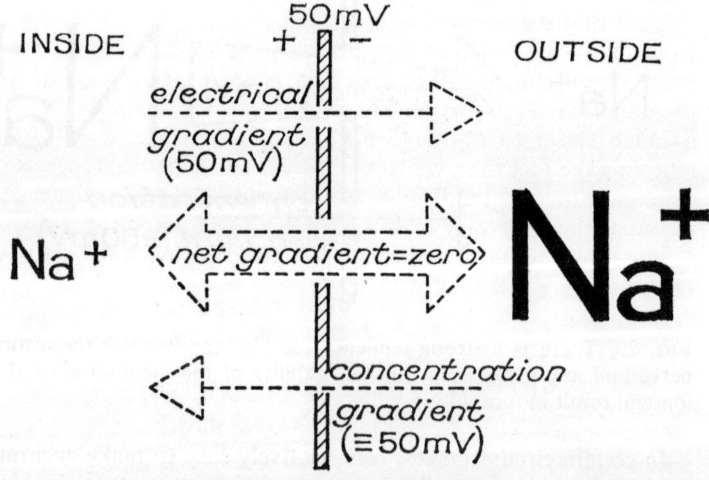

FIG. 26. The Na-influx which follows a rise in P_{Na} will reverse membrane potential and eventually generate an electrical gradient which curtails further Na-gain. Thus, a new equilibrium condition will be achieved in which the concentration gradient is exactly balanced by the new electrical gradient. Since these Na-currents involve only a minute fraction of the total number of Na ions available, the concentration gradient will remain at its resting level and equilibrium will be achieved when the electrical gradient has reached an equivalent value, i.e. when membrane potential has reached E_{Na} (calculated from the resting Na concentration gradient).

exactly balances the concentration gradient (E_{Na}) and hence $E_m = E_{Na} = +50$ mV.

Similarly, if the membrane became permeable to K ions only, membrane potential would shift towards E_K (-75 mV). In general, any rise in permeability involving only one ion will tend to shift membrane potential towards the equilibrium potential for that ion. (These predictions are made on the assumption that concentration gradients *remain at their resting levels*, whence the equilibrium potentials can be calculated from the resting concentration gradients. If the ionic currents involved an appreciable proportion of the available ions, then concentration gradients would also change along with the membrane potential and it would no longer be possible to make simple predictions from conditions in the quiescent nerve.)

Unfortunately, the situation in the squid axon is complicated by the fact that the membrane is rarely permeable to only one ion. Even so, a knowledge of the various equilibrium potentials can prove very useful, as will be seen in subsequent chapters. For the present, it is interesting to note that the resting potential (-60 mV) is much closer to E_K (-75 mV) than it is to E_{Na} ($+50$ mV), reflecting the fact that, whilst permeable to both ions, the resting membrane favours the K ions. It can also be seen that membrane potential can only vary within the range -75 mV (permeable to K ions only) to $+50$ mV (permeable to Na ions only) and its value at any given time within these limits will reflect the ratio $P_K : P_{Na}$.

CHAPTER 3

The Nerve Impulse

The nerve impulse is a wave of electrical activity which propagates along the axon without decrement. Fig. 27 shows an intracellular recording from a squid giant axon and illustrates the reversal of membrane potential, from its resting level of −60 mV, to a peak of +45 mV during the impulse. The main spike has a

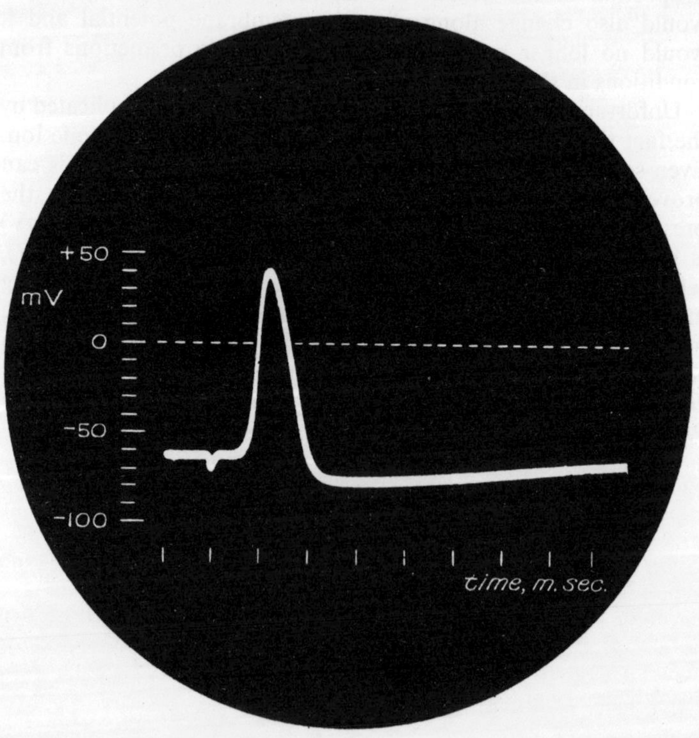

FIG. 27. A nerve impulse recorded with an internal electrode from the isolated axon of squid. The membrane potential is about − 60mV during rest and reverses during the action potential, almost reaching + 50mV. (Hodgkin, 1958.)

duration of about 1 millisecond and is followed by a prolonged hyperpolarization* lasting several milliseconds.

Experimentally, the most convenient way of generating such impulses in the axon is by passing a brief electric current across the membrane. However, not all currents lead to the generation of nerve impulses, and in part, the form of the recording depends upon the position of the pick-up electrodes relative to the site of stimulation. It can be seen from Fig. 28 that nerve impulses are only initiated by depolarizing currents, and then, only when E_m is

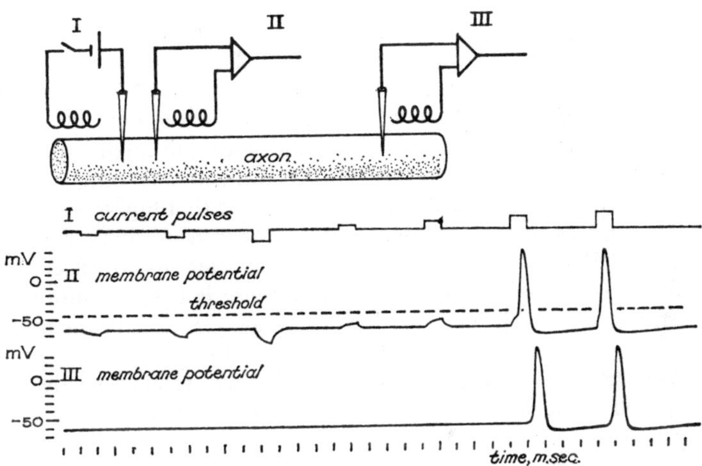

FIG. 28. The effect of passing current pulses across the nerve membrane (trace I) on the membrane potential of the nerve axon recorded locally (trace II) and at a distance (trace III). It can be seen that such stimulation always gives rise to local electrotonic potentials, but propagating action potentials only arise after depolarization of the membrane beyond a certain threshold. The local responses are of a kind that can be recorded from any transmission cable, but the self-reinforcing action potentials are unique to nerve and muscle and derive from special features in the membrane.

*In the resting state, with a steady potential difference between the inside and outside of the cell, the nerve membrane separates positive and negative charges and is therefore said to be *polarized*. When the membrane potential is increased, then the charge separation is also raised and the membrane is said to be *hyper*polarized. If the membrane potential is reduced, the membrane is said to be *de*polarized.

driven beyond a certain threshold level—in Fig. 28, at about 15 mV depolarization. However, the recordings made close to the site of stimulation reveal that all applied currents have a *local* effect on the membrane potential. Clearly, when adequate, depolarization brings about some change in the neurone which converts it from a mere passive cable into an impulse-generating device. The local changes in E_m—called *electrotonic potentials*—are due simply to the redistribution of charges across the membrane capacitance in accordance with the electric field impressed by the stimulator. Such potentials are particularly noticeable with hyperpolarizing currents since they are never obscured by impulses. The magnitude of the electrotonic potentials is a function of the intensity of the applied field and the passive cable properties of the axon. Currents spread from the stimulating electrodes into the adjacent region of the axon but the high longitudinal resistance encountered causes a rapid attenuation of these potentials and they are hardly measureable only a few millimeters away. It should be clear from this that high-resistance cables such as nerves, can only be used for transmitting information if the signals are boosted at regular intervals to offset the severe attenuation. Thus, the nerve impulse is a self-reinforcing phenomenon which draws upon the energy resources of the axon as it invades each successive segment.

The term "electrotonic potentials" thus refers strictly to localized electrical disturbances and though not actually part of the nerve impulse proper, these potentials are very important in the transmission of the impulse from one point on the axon to the next. Since membrane potential is reversed in the region of the impulse, the latter will exchange ions with the neighbouring areas of the axon i.e. *local circuit currents* will flow between the adjacent "active" and "inactive" regions of the axon. As a result of these currents, the quiescent membrane immediately ahead of the nerve impulse is depolarized to threshold, triggering changes in the membrane which will generate an impulse there. In this way, the impulse invades successive segments of the axon.

Permeability Changes Associated with the Nerve Impulse

During the nerve impulse, membrane potential reverses and approaches E_{Na}, suggesting that the main spike is due to a rapid influx of Na ions presumeably following upon a transient rise in the permeability of the membrane to this ion. Hodgkin & Katz

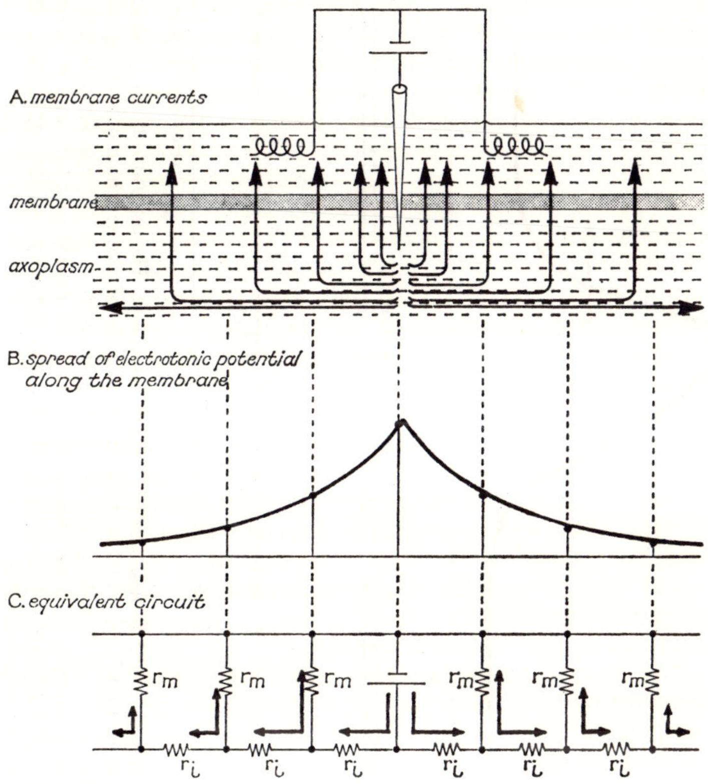

FIG. 29. The spread of local circuit currents and their electrotonic potentials along the axon. A: The spatial distribution of the currents flowing from an intracellular stimulating electrode at a given instant in time. B: The magnitude of the electrotonic potential at various points along the axon at that same instant. C: An equivalent electrical circuit for the nerve axon, where r_m = membrane resistance per unit area, and r_l = internal (or longitudinal) resistance per unit length. The axon can be regarded as a passive resistive cable and the longitudinal current travelling through the axoplasm diminishes progressively with distance as it leaks out through the membrane. Thus, the electrotonic potential decays exponentially with increasing distance and in actual nerves it is rare for them to penetrate more than a few millimetres along the axon.

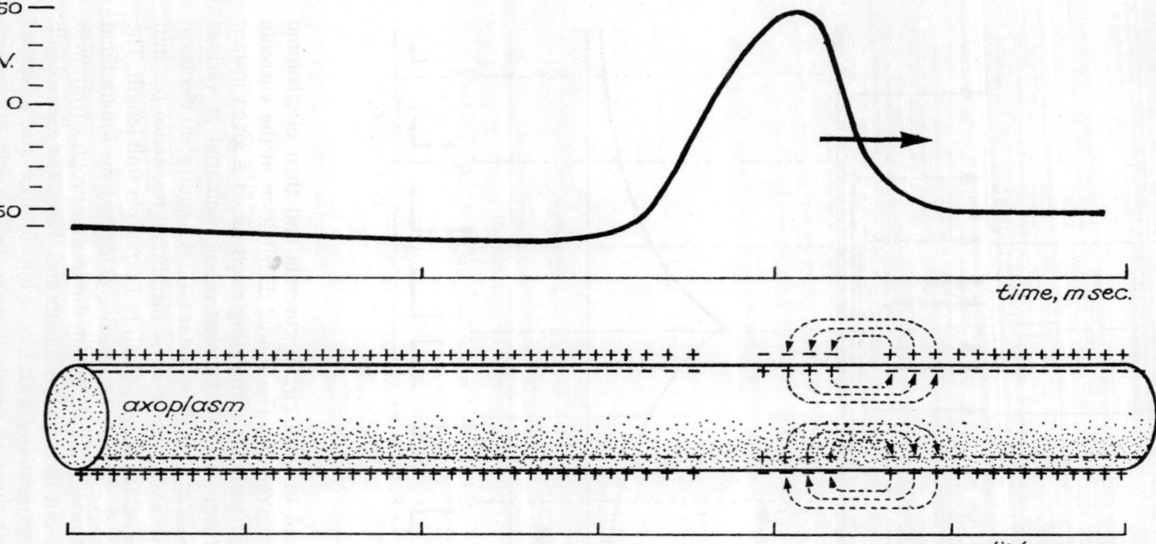

FIG. 30. The role of the local circuit currents in the propagation of the nerve impulse. The diagram shows a voltage profile of an activated axon at a given instant in time and indicates the exchange of charge which occurs between adjacent active and inactive regions. As a result of these local circuit currents, a decremental wave of depolarization travels in the vanguard of the impulse and activates each successive segment of the membrane. Information transmission along nerve axons takes the form of explosive impulses which travel the length of the axon somewhat in the manner of a flame traversing a trail of gunpowder.

(1949) provided strong evidence in support of this view when they found that the amplitude of the spike could be reduced by replacing some of the Na ions in the external solution with a "neutral" substance such as dextrose. Reducing the $[Na]_o$ clearly reduces the concentration gradient driving Na ions into the axon, hence lowering E_{Na} and so curtailing the excursion in

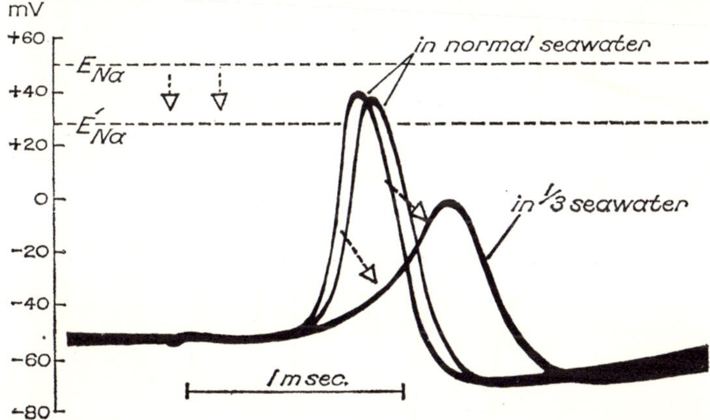

FIG. 31. The effect of removing some of the Na ions from the bathing medium on the form of the action potential. Replacing two thirds of the seawater with isotonic dextrose produced a marked reduction in the amplitude of the action potential which was in accord with the calculated drop in E_{Na} (to E'_{Na}). The dextrose molecules are too large to penetrate the membrane and hence could not contribute towards the action currents. (After Hodgkin & Katz, 1949.)

membrane potential (see Fig. 31). As might be expected, a rise in $[Na]_o$ produces an increase in the amplitude of the impulse.

After the main spike, the membrane repolarizes but overshoots the resting level and approaches E_K. Thus, after discriminating heavily in favour of Na ions, the activated membrane now switches its preference over to the K ions. However, two features of this repolarization seem to indicate that it is something more than a mere return to the resting condition: the high speed with which it is accomplished, and the "overshoot". These factors suggest that the initial rise in P_{Na} is followed closely by a considerable rise in P_K so that the repolarizing membrane discrimi-

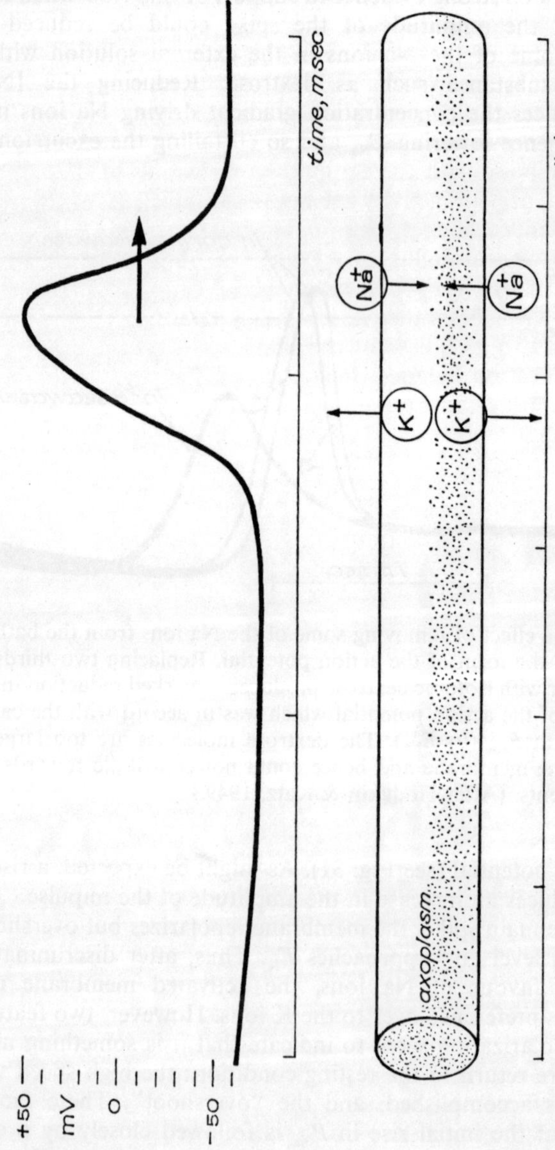

FIG. 32. The major ionic movements generating the nerve impulse are a rapid influx of Na ions (depolarization) closely followed by an efflux of K ions (repolarization).

nates even more heavily in favour of the K ions than the resting membrane. If this is the case, then the depolarizing, Na-influx should be followed by a hyperpolarizing, K-efflux. Tracer experiments have shown that nervous activity is indeed associated with a net leakage of K ions from the axon (Keynes, 1951a).

Thus, by simply correlating the changes in E_m which make up the nerve impulse with the equilibrium potentials of the various ions present, nervous activity becomes explicable entirely in terms of permeability changes. An initial brief rise in P_{Na}, which permits a transient influx of cations (Na) and reverses E_m, is followed by a rise in P_K with an attendant cation loss (K) which repolarizes the membrane. A few milliseconds later, the membrane returns to its quiescent condition and the exchange pump restores the cation balance. It is assumed that the permeability changes are triggered by the depolarization associated with the local circuit currents.

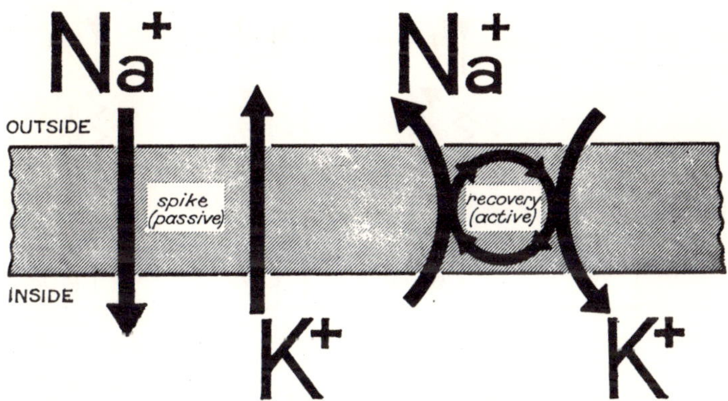

FIG. 33. The activity cycle of the excitable nerve membrane. The action potential results entirely from passive Na- and K-fluxes which follow changes in membrane permeability. During the subsequent recovery period, the cation balance is restored by a pump which derives its energy from cellular metabolism. (After Hodgkin & Keynes, 1955a.)

In recent years, the properties of the nerve membrane have been the subject of intensive research. As a result of these studies, it is now possible to reconstruct a much more complete account of the fundamental mechanisms underlying nervous activity. Before considering these recent developments, it is necessary to quantify some of the parameters which, thus far, have only been considered qualitatively. In particular, it is essential to be clear about the parameters which must be recorded in order to make accurate estimates of membrane permeability. The simplest way of doing this is by constructing an electrical model of the membrane.

An Electrical Model of the Nerve Membrane

The membrane can be regarded as a "leaky" capacitance, which under resting conditions allows small currents to flow through it. In the model, these currents move through separate Na-, K- and Cl-channels and each has its own chemical gradient

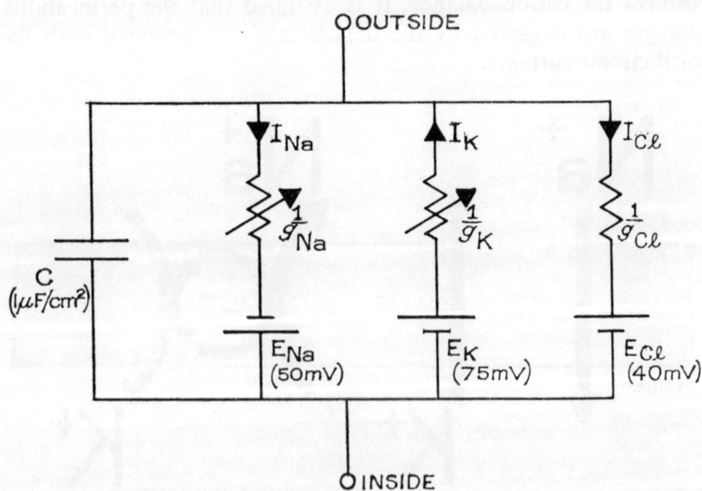

FIG. 34. An electrical model of the excitable nerve membrane. The potential difference across the membrane capacitance (C) can be altered by the passage of charges along any one of the three ionic channels. (The transient passive currents which accompany any change in membrane conductance are several hundred times greater than those carried by the ionic pumps. Thus, it may take a second or more for the pumps to restore the ionic balance after a single impulse whose duration is a mere millisecond. Clearly, the passive currents under consideration here are large enough for us to be able to ignore any effects of the pumps, at least in the short term.) (Model after Hodgkin & Huxley, 1952d.)

(represented by the equilibrium potential for the ion) and variable resistance. An increase in the permeability of the membrane to a particular ion corresponds to a drop in the resistance of the channel concerned. Such a change would allow the ion to flow down its electrochemical gradient, charging the membrane capacity up to E_{ion}.

However, biologists in the main find the inverse relationship between permeability and resistance inconvenient and prefer to use the "reciprocal-ohm" or conductance:

$$\text{permeability} \propto \frac{1}{\text{resistance}}$$

and

$$\text{conductance} = \frac{1}{\text{resistance}}.$$

Whence

$$\text{permeability} \propto \text{conductance}.$$

Thus, the electrical analogue of permeability which will be used here is conductance.

From Ohm's Law

$$\text{resistance} = \frac{\text{potential difference}}{\text{current}}.$$

Whence

$$\text{conductance} = \frac{\text{current}}{\text{potential difference}}.$$

This simple equation defines the permeability of the membrane (i.e. its conductance) in terms of the current flowing per unit potential difference, and can be extended to accommodate the situation in the nerve axon:

$$\text{conductance for a given ion } (g_{\text{ion}}) = \frac{\text{ionic current } (I_{\text{ion}})}{\text{net driving force on the ion}}.$$

However

net driving force on the ion

$$= \text{electrochemical gradient on the ion}$$
$$= E_m - E_{\text{ion}} \text{ (see p.19).}$$

Thus, in general

$$g_{\text{ion}} = \frac{I_{\text{ion}}}{E_m - E_{\text{ion}}}.$$

This equation can now be applied to each of the ions involved, and defines their individual conductances:

$$g_{Na} = \frac{I_{Na}}{E_m - E_{Na}}; \quad g_K = \frac{I_K}{E_m - E_K}; \quad g_{Cl} = \frac{I_{Cl}}{E_m - E_{Cl}}.$$

Having derived a precise definition to describe the permeability function of the membrane, it can now be seen that further studies in this field must attempt simultaneous measurements of the individual ionic currents and their electrochemical gradients. During the nerve impulse, changes in membrane permeability produce both varying currents and gradients so that the effects of the one tend to obscure the effects of the other and vice versa. So far, we have only been able to describe the permeability changes accompanying nervous activity in very general terms because we have had to base all of our deductions on measurements of membrane potential alone. In order to establish firm data about the permeability function, a slightly different approach is needed.

It was shown earlier (p. 14 *et seq.*), that the passive exchange of ions between the cell and its surroundings is determined by the permeability of the membrane and the net driving force on the ions. This can now be stated in precise, mathematical terms:

Rearranging the general permeability equation—

$$I_{ion} = g_{ion} . (E_m - E_{ion}).$$

It will be apparent from this expression, that if the ionic currents could be measured whilst the electrochemical gradients were held steady i.e. E_m and E_{ion} were constant, then these currents could be a reliable monitor of membrane conductance changes:

$$I_{ion} = g_{ion} . (a\ constant).$$
$$\text{i.e. } I_{ion} \propto g_{ion}.$$

Cole developed a method, now known as the *voltage clamp* technique, which can be used to adjust the membrane potential to any desired level and then hold it steady (Cole, 1949). The initial procedure involves depolarization of the membrane beyond threshold to trigger the permeability changes which would normally lead to the development of an impulse. However, the subsequent ionic currents are not allowed to generate an impulse, the charges being led off by a feedback amplifier, so that E_m remains "clamped" at a new level. This means that the permeability changes associated with the impulse will proceed in the absence of any potential changes (though they will take a somewhat modified form). Since the equilibrium potentials for the various ions can be assumed to remain virtually unchanged by any transient ionic currents (p. 31 *et seq.*), maintaining a steady E_m will ensure a constant driving force on the ions i.e. $E_m - E_{ion}$ = a constant. Fluctuations in the ionic currents during such clamps must therefore result from conductance changes which, under normal, unclamped conditions, would yield a nerve impulse. It is a simple matter to record these currents and use them to calculate the time course of the underlying conductance changes:

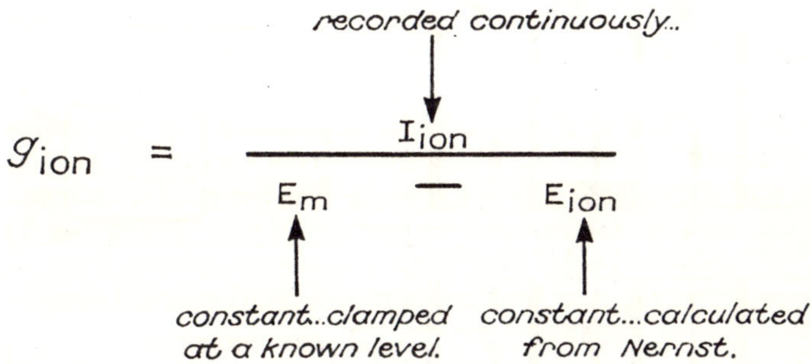

FIG. 35. A simple schema to show the basis of the voltage clamp approach to the study of permeability changes.

The voltage clamp technique can thus be used to deduce the sequence of conductance changes which accompany activation of the membrane. By varying the level of the clamp voltage, it is possible to investigate the relationship between membrane conductance and membrane potential. We shall see that the dependence of permeability on E_m is a subtle one and plays a crucial role in the production of the nerve impulse.

The ionic currents which are recorded during voltage clamps and from which permeabilities will be calculated, reflect the total net ionic exchange across the membrane and hence no distinction is made between the different ionic species contributing towards this total. Of course, there are two ions involved in these permeability changes—Na and K ions. For this reason, it has been necessary to devise techniques for the separation of the total ionic currents into its separate components—I_{Na} and I_K—from which it is then possible to estimate the individual conductances—g_{Na} and g_K.

Voltage Clamp Studies

Voltage clamp studies have made a major contribution to our understanding of nervous activity. Prominent amongst the many publications in this field are the papers of Hodgkin & Huxley, who gathered sufficient quantitative material to formulate a

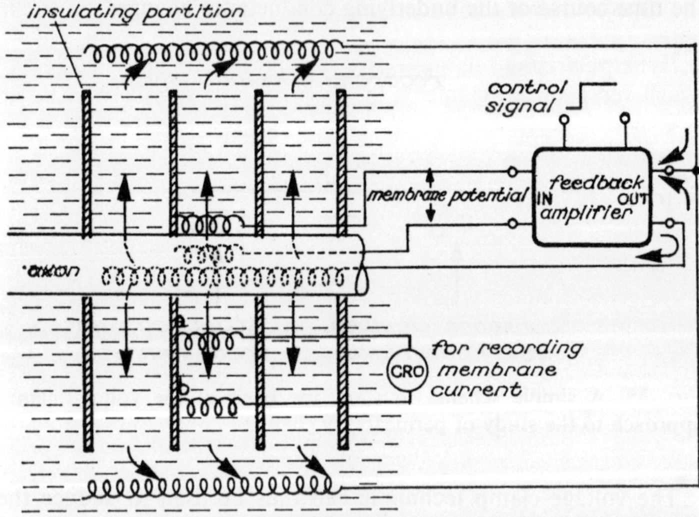

FIG. 36. The voltage clamp technique is used to depolarize the nerve membrane to some new level and then hold it steady. The permeability changes which follow this activation of the membrane proceed in a modified form, but the impulse proper, i.e. the action potential, which normally accompanies them, is absent. In these special circumstances, the excursions in membrane permeability can be followed simply by recording the membrane currents. The feedback amplifier senses the membrane potential at its input and supplies output currents which bring this input into line with the control voltage. In this way, the experimenter is able to specify membrane potential by manipulating the control signal. Note that the guard system ensures radial current flow across a measured area of the membrane and that the net magnitude of these currents in the innermost compartment is monitored via electrodes "a" and "b".

mathematical description of the events which make up the nerve impulse (Hodgkin & Huxley, 1952a,b,c,d; Hodgkin, Huxley & Katz, 1952). These important experiments will be our main concern for the remainder of this chapter.

The experimental arrangements are shown diagrammatically in Fig. 36. Isolated squid axons were used because their very considerable size makes it possible to introduce electrodes and perform other manipulations. The feedback amplifier supplied the currents necessary to alter membrane potential in a stepwise fashion and the ionic currents moving across a restricted area of the membrane were recorded using electrodes "a" and "b" in the bath.

Hyperpolarizing clamps produce graded inward currents* which represent adjustments in the resting leakage currents due

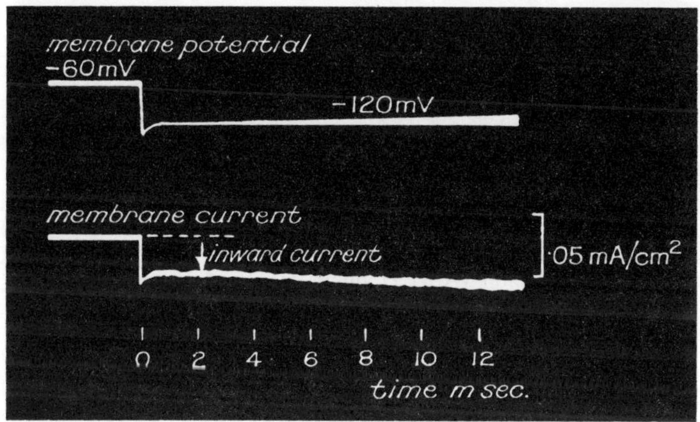

FIG. 37. The membrane currents during a hyperpolarizing clamp in a squid axon. Note that the currents recorded in these voltage clamp experiments are always the total net current (with inward current always producing a downward deflection of the beam). The numbers over the voltage records indicate the membrane potential in mV. (After Hodgkin, Huxley & Katz, 1952.)

*In refering to the ionic currents across the membrane, it is conventional to indicate the direction of the net *positive* current. Thus, inward currents involve a net influx of positive current which could be carried by an influx of cations and/or an efflux of anions.

solely to the change in the driving force on the ions. Most of the current is carried by K ions, the rise in E_m favouring further K-influx.

With small depolarizing clamps—of less than 15 mV—the ionic balance is disturbed in favour of an increased K-efflux, leading to graded outward currents.

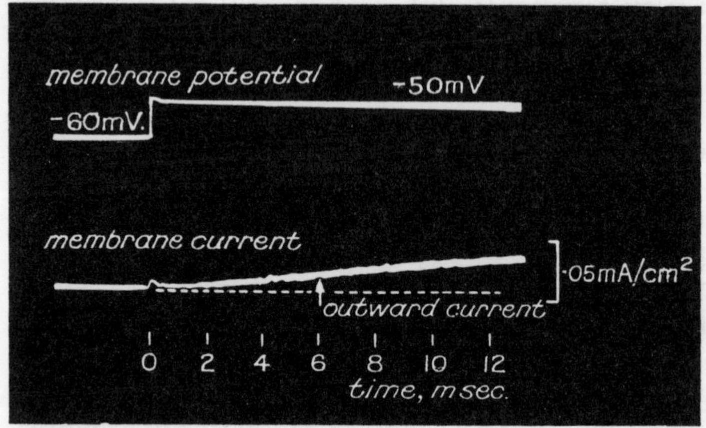

FIG. 38. The membrane currents during a subthreshold depolarizing clamp in a squid axon. (After Hodgkin, Huxley & Katz, 1952.)

Thus far, no permeability changes need be invoked to explain the results and the membrane remains in its quiescent condition throughout the clamps. However, when the depolarization exceeeds 15 mV, the pattern of membrane currents becomes more complex and can only be explained by assuming changes in the permeability of the membrane. You will recollect that 15 mV is the threshold depolarization which must be exceeded to trigger impulse activity in the axon. The clear suggestion here is that the permeability changes associated with supra-threshold clamps are probably concerned in some way with activation of the membrane. In general, the membrane currents during these clamps consist of two components—an initial, inward current of brief duration, rapidly followed by a prolonged outward current. The nature, magnitude and time relations of these ionic currents accord very closely with those postulated earlier to account for the nerve impulse i.e. a brief inward surge (of Na ions) followed by a more prolonged outward flux (of K ions). This is very encouraging

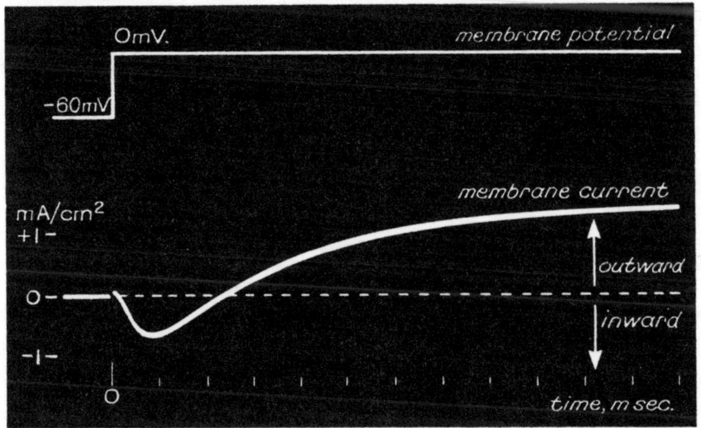

FIG. 39. The membrane currents during a suprathreshold depolarizing clamp in a squid axon consist of a transient wave of inward current followed by a maintained outward current. (After Hodgkin, Huxley & Katz, 1952.)

since it suggests that the voltage clamp experiments involve the very same mechanisms which, in the unclamped nerve, would generate the impulse. If this can be proved, then the technique becomes a valuable source of information concerning the properties of the activated membrane. Before proceeding any further, it is necessary to establish the identity of the ions which carry the currents during the voltage clamps.

The "Early" Current. If the initial surge of current is carried by Na ions, then certain predictions can be made about its magnitude and direction at various clamp voltages. Thus, its direction should be determined wholly by the electrochemical gradient on the Na ions, which is a function of E_m and E_{Na}. Since $E_{Na} = +50$ mV, it would be expected that clamping the axon at +50 mV—a depolarization of some 110 mV—would completely abolish the "early" current. For smaller depolarizations, the net driving force would be negative, producing an inward current, whilst for greater depolarizations the net driving force would be positive and the current outward. This reversal of the initial current can best be illustrated by considering three simple examples:

1. A depolarizing clamp of 70 mV would change E_m from its resting level of -60 mV to $+10$ mV.

Net driving force on the Na ions

$$= (E_m - E_{Na})\text{mV}$$
$$= (+10) - (+50)\text{mV}$$
$$= -40 \text{ mV}.$$

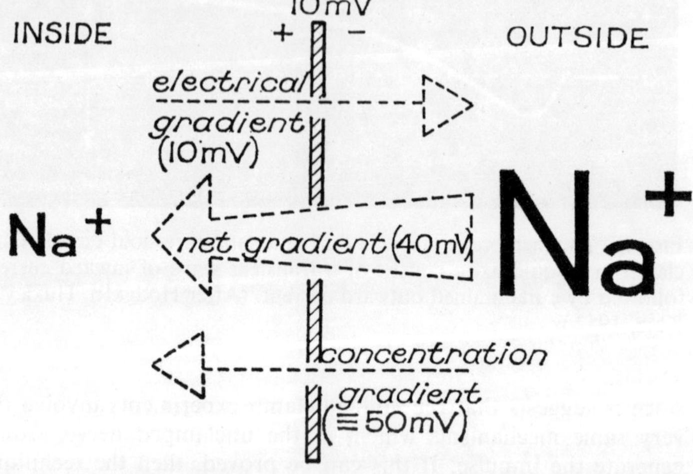

FIG. 40. The electrochemical forces on the Na ions in the squid axon during a voltage clamp which shifts membrane potential to + 10mV.

Thus, there would be a *net inward current* of Na ions, which would decrease progressively as the clamp voltage approaches E_{Na}.

2. A depolarizing clamp of 110 mV would change E_m from its resting level of -60 mV to $+50$ mV (i.e. E_{Na}).

Net driving force on the Na ions

$$= (E_m - E_{Na})\text{mV}$$
$$= (+50) - (+50)\text{mV}$$
$$= 0 \text{ mV}.$$

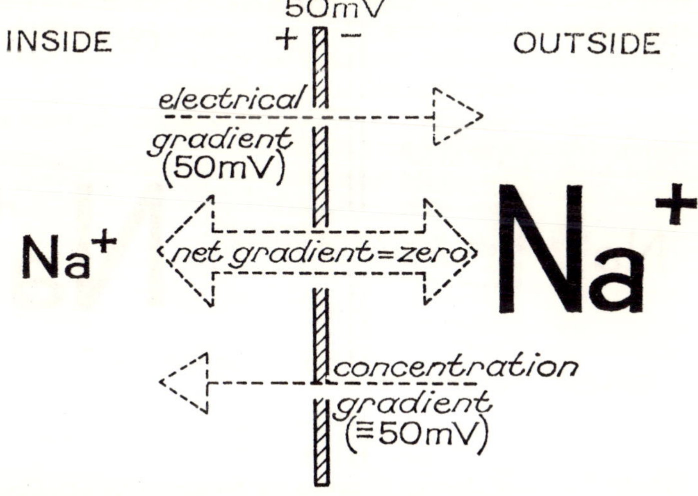

FIG. 41. The electrochemical forces on the Na ions in the squid axon during a voltage clamp which shifts membrane potential to + 50mV.

Thus, the Na ion is equilibrated so that there would be *no net current.*

3. A depolarizing clamp of 150 mV would change E_m from its resting level of -60 mV to $+90$ mV.

Net driving force on the Na ions

$$\begin{aligned} &= (E_m - E_{Na})\text{mV} \\ &= (+90) - (+50)\text{mV} \\ &= +40 \text{ mV}. \end{aligned}$$

Thus, there would be a *net outward current* of Na ions.

Hodgkin & Huxley performed a series of voltage clamps and found that the initial current did in fact reverse at a membrane potential very close to E_{Na}. Clearly, these results only become meaningful if we assume that an early result of depolarization is an increase in g_{Na}. The net current carried by the Na ions is only inward so long as the depolarization is strong enough to increase g_{Na}, but not strong enough to make E_m sufficiently positive to overcome the concentration gradient. The critical value for E_m when equilibrium conditions prevail is called *the reversal potential*

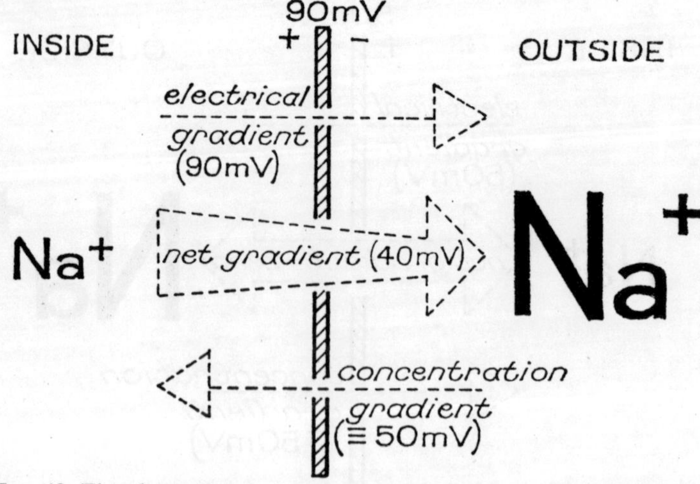

FIG. 42. The electrochemical forces on the Na ions in the squid axon during a voltage clamp which shifts membrane potential to + 90mV.

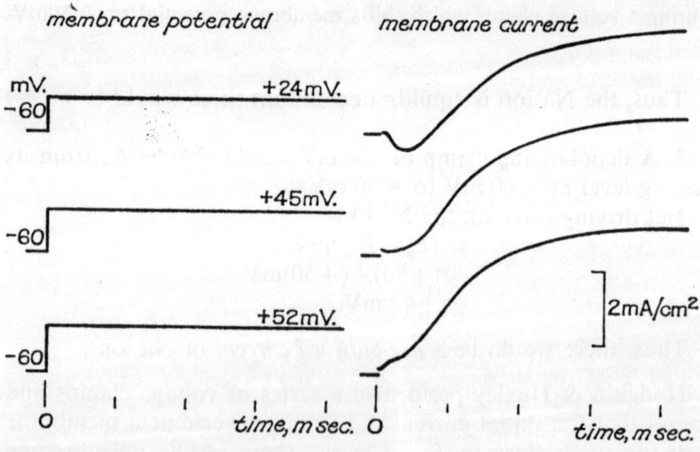

FIG. 43. The reversal potential for the "early" current in the squid axon. The initial surge of inward current which usually accompanies depolarizing clamps (see top trace) is virtually absent at a potential of + 45mV (middle trace) and actually reversed at + 52mV (bottom trace). Thus, the reversal of the "early" current occurs at a membrane potential very close to E_{Na}(+ 50mV), strongly suggesting that this current is carried by Na ions. (After Hodgkin & Huxley, 1952a.)

for the "early" current. The fact that this reversal potential corresponds to E_{Na} is the central piece of evidence for the view that Na ions carry the "early" current. In a further series of experiments, Hodgkin & Huxley removed any possible doubts about the essential validity of this case. Thus, they repeated these voltage clamps in low-sodium solutions and found that the reversal potential for the "early" current always reduced in exact accordance with the estimated reduction in E_{Na}.

The "Delayed" Current. The outward current which arises with a delay after depolarization is unaffected by changing $[Na]_o$. This finding is consistent with the hypothesis put forward earlier that the "delayed" current involves those mechanisms responsible for the falling phase of the impulse i.e. a rise in g_K. One way of putting this hypothesis to the test is to see if the "delayed" current has a reversal potential which approximates to E_K. However, the estimated value for E_K in the squid axon is -75 mV, which means that if the "delayed" current is carried by K ions its reversal potential can only be reached by hyperpolarizing the membrane. It has already been seen that hyperpolarizing clamps are not accompanied by permeability changes, the axon remaining in its *quiescent* condition. We are only concerned here with the permeability characteristics of the *activated* membrane and this condition can only be achieved by depolarizing the axon. In order to circumvent this difficulty, Hodgkin & Huxley made use of the fact that the changes in membrane permeability which accompany depolarizing clamps not only take time to develop, but also take time to decay when the clamp is removed. Thus, the permeability changes established *during* the depolarizing clamp persist for a short time *after* repolarization of the membrane. Repolarization can be used to provide a new driving force for the ions and, for a brief period, currents will flow through channels which have remained open since the period of depolarization. Clearly, repolarization will result in an immediate surge of current (due to the residual conductance) whose direction is determined entirely by the net driving force on the ions concerned i.e. it will be a function of E_m on repolarization. In their experiments, Hodgkin & Huxley applied depolarizing clamps to trigger the normal permeability changes in the membrane, and each time when the "delayed" current was established, repolarized the axon to various levels around E_K.

The "tail" of current following repolarization during the

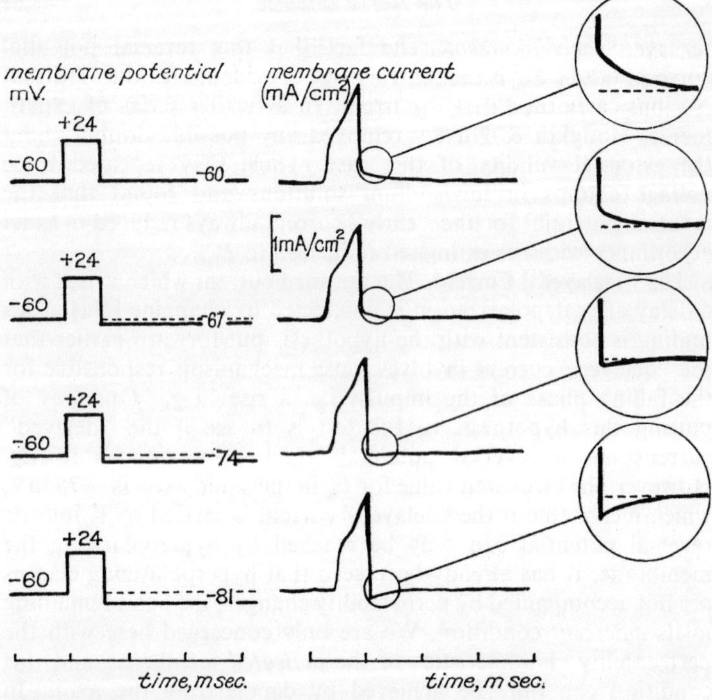

FIG. 44. The reversal potential for the "delayed" current in the squid axon. Sudden repolarization during the "delayed" current is accompanied by a brief "tail" of current due to residual permeability in the membrane. Thus, the "delayed" current persists for a few milliseconds after repolarization. If it is assumed that the channels which carry the "delayed" current also carry the "tail" of current—which seems a reasonable assumption—then clearly they will share the same reversal potential. Confining our attention to the "tail" of current, the top two traces reveal that its direction is normally outward and causes a delay in the return of the membrane current to its resting level. However, as the interior of the axon is subsequently made more negative on repolarization then the "tail" of current reverses to a surge of inward current (lower two traces). In order to display these repolarization currents more clearly, they are shown at ten times higher gain in the insets. It can be seen that the reversal potential for these repolarization currents is somewhere between − 67mV and −, 74mV, i.e. very close to E_K (− 75mV) and providing strong indirect evidence for the view that the "delayed" current is carried by K ions. (Note that this experiment was done in low-Na seawater so that the initial current is reversed throughout, i.e. outward.) (After Hodgkin & Huxley, 1952b.)

"delayed" current was outward at the resting potential and was reversed when E_m exceeded this by more than 12 mV. We can conclude from this that the reversal potential for the "delayed" current is about -72 mV, a value which compares very favourably with E_K and confirms the idea that the "delayed" current is carried by K ions.

Separation of the Ionic Current into I_{Na} and I_K. The above experiments show that, in the main, the "early" current is carried by Na ions and the "delayed" current by K ions. These currents

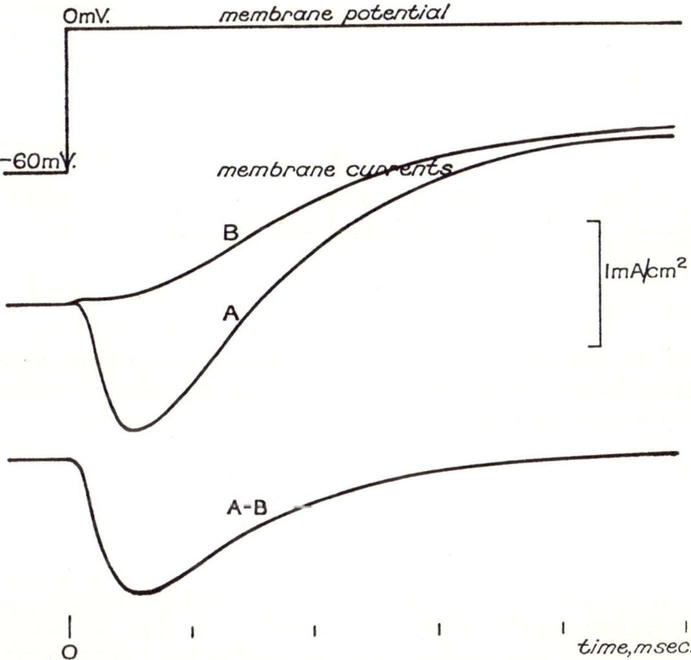

FIG. 45. Separation of the total ionic current into the components carried by Na and K ions. Trace A: shows the characteristic membrane currents for a depolarization of 60mV. Trace B: shows a repetition of the previous experiment after reducing $[Na]_0$ so that the Na ions are equilibrated throughout the clamp, i.e. E_{Na} is reduced to 0mV. Since the Na ions are now equilibrated, only the K currents are recorded. Curve A-B: is a plot of the Na current during the clamp, obtained by subtraction of trace B from trace A. (Hodgkin, 1958.)

must follow increases in g_{Na} and g_K which are in general, out of phase, but it is not possible from the present results to separate the total current into its two components with any great accuracy. In particular, it is not clear to what extent the changes in g_{Na} and g_K overlap. This difficulty can only be resolved by devising some method which will separate the total ionic current into its two components, I_{Na} and I_K. The approach employed by Hodgkin & Huxley was based on the principle that when the axon is clamped at E_{Na}, all the I_{Na} is selectively abolished since the Na ions are equilibrated, and any recorded currents must be carried by K ions.

Trace "A" in Fig. 45 shows the familiar pattern of membrane currents which result for a depolarizing clamp of 60 mV (shifting E_m from its resting level of -60 mV to 0 mV). For curve "B", this clamp was repeated after first reducing E_{Na} to 0 mV by an appropriate reduction in the external Na ion concentration. Curve "B" thus represents the K-currents only since the Na ions have been equilibrated. Curve "A–B" is a plot of the Na-currents obtained simply by subtracting curve "B" from curve "A":

$$\text{total ionic current} = I = I_{Na} + I_K.$$

Whence

$$I_{Na} = I - I_K.$$

This analysis of the membrane currents during voltage clamps has recently received pharmacological confirmation through the use of two drugs, tetrodotoxin (TTX) and tetraethylammonium (TEA). Voltage clamp studies on axons poisoned with these drugs resolve the currents into two separate components which show

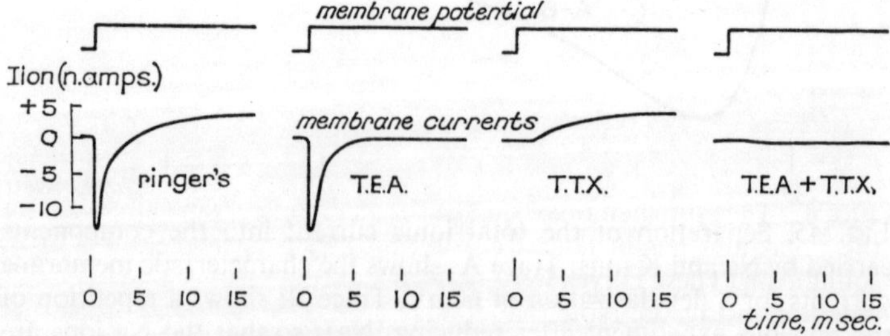

FIG. 46. Membrane currents during suprathreshold depolarizing clamps in frog myelinated nerve fibre in the presence of various drugs. Note the suppression of the late (potassium-) current by TEA, and of the early (sodium-) current by TTX. (After Hille, 1967.)

a very marked similarity to the Na- and K-currents described by Hodgkin & Huxley (Moore, Blaustein, Anderson & Narahashi, 1967; Hille, 1967). TEA-poisoned axons show only the "early" currents, whilst axons treated with TTX only generate the "delayed" currents. Such a close correspondence between the results of two studies which employ such widely differing techniques could hardly be fortuitous, and gives very strong support to Hodgkin & Huxley's analysis. The pharmacological data also reinforces the view that different ions move through different channels in the membrane.

Conductance Changes During Voltage Clamps. Having determined the time course of I_{Na} and I_K during voltage clamps, we now have sufficient information to estimate g_{Na} and g_K, as functions of time, from the equations:

$$g_{Na} = \frac{I_{Na}}{E_m - E_{Na}} \quad \text{and} \quad g_K = \frac{I_K}{E_m - E_K}.$$

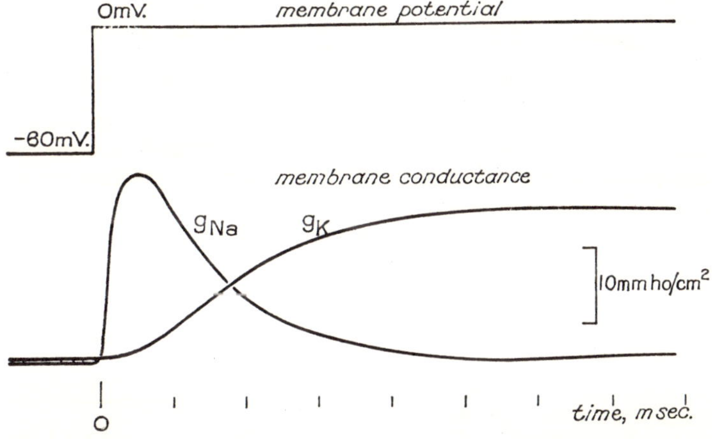

FIG. 47. The estimated time course of the sodium conductance (g_{Na}) and the potassium conductance (g_K) during a depolarizing clamp in the squid axon. These curves were derived from those in Fig. 45 using the equation in Fig. 35. Note that conductance is measured in "reciprocal ohms" or mhos. (Hodgkin, 1958.)

It is clear from Fig. 47 that the rise in g_{Na} is an early, transient effect of depolarization, whilst the increase in g_K takes much

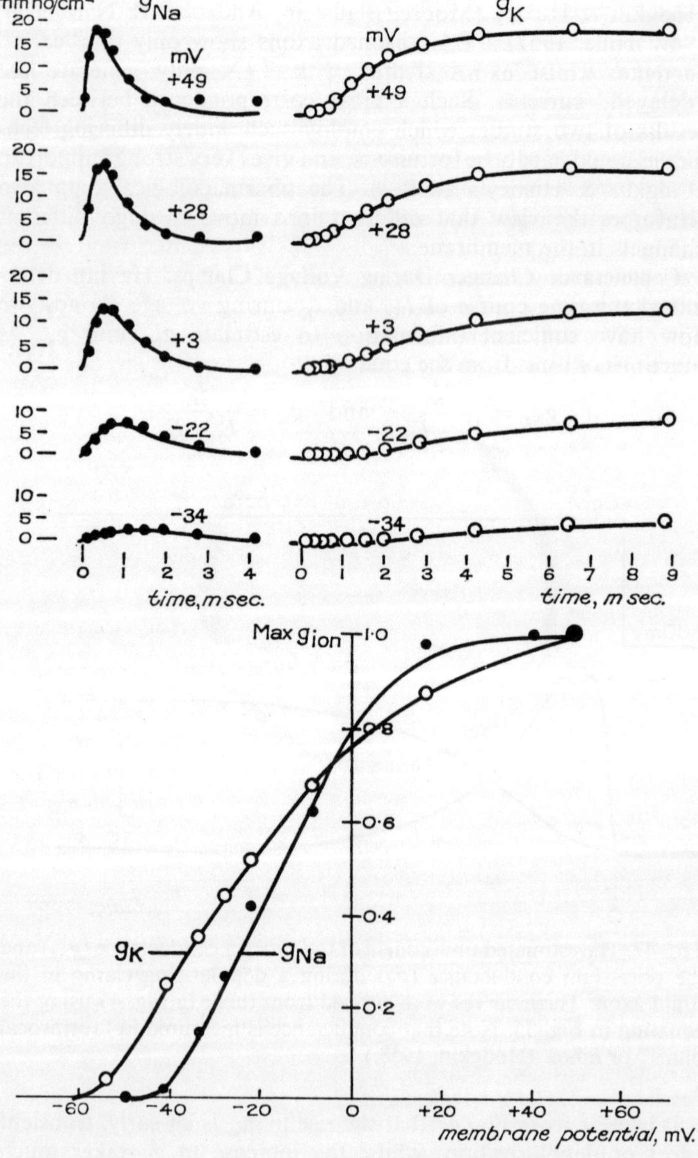

mmho/cm²
g_{Na}
g_K
mV
+49
+28
+3
−22
−34
20
15
10
5
0
0 1 2 3 4
time, msec.
0 1 2 3 4 5 6 7 8 9
time, m sec.
Max g_{ion}
1·0
0·8
0·6
0·4
0·2
g_K
g_{Na}
−60 −40 −20 0 +20 +40 +60
membrane potential, mV.

longer to develop and persists for as long as the clamp is maintained.

By repeating these experiments at different membrane voltages, Hodgkin & Huxley found that g_{Na} and g_K were also dependent upon the strength of depolarization. Thus, over the normal working range of membrane potentials, both g_{Na} and g_K increase as the strength of depolarization increases. Some such relationship could have been anticipated from what we already know about the importance of depolarization in the initiation of the impulse.

The voltage dependence of g_{Na} provides an explanation for the very steep rising phase of the nerve impulse: depolarization of the axon by local circuit currents raises g_{Na} which allows Na ions to enter the axon causing further depolarization etc. This cycle of events, in which E_m and g_{Na} reinforce one another, results in E_m

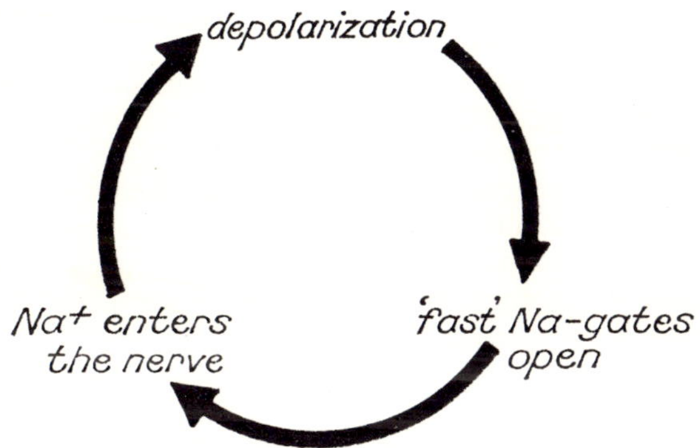

FIG. 49. The dependence of the sodium conductance on membrane potential results in a positive feedback cycle which generates the steep rising phase of the action potential. (After Hodgkin, 1964.)

FIG. 48. The dependence of membrane conductance on the membrane potential. Above: The estimated time course of g_{Na} and g_K for different displacements of membrane potential. The numbers on each curve denote the membrane potential (in mV) during the clamp. (Hodgkin, 1958.) Below: Maximum g_{Na} and g_K reached during voltage clamps of varying intensities. (Maxima are calculated relative to the value reached at + 60mV.) Note particularly the steep curve for sodium, which helps to explain the brisk rise in g_{Na} following depolarizations of 15mV or more. (Replotted from data of Hodgkin & Huxley, 1952a.)

moving rapidly towards E_{Na} before the "delayed" effects of depolarization (increased g_K) have had time to develop.

Inactivation of the Sodium Channels. The experiments discussed so far do not explain why the g_{Na} (unlike the g_K) declines from its peak back to the resting level during prolonged clamps. Why is the rise in g_{Na} so short-lived despite the continuance of the clamp? Further voltage clamp studies showed that E_m exerts a dual effect on g_{Na}.

When depolarizing clamps follow a conditioning period of depolarization, the subsequent Na-currents (and therefore also g_{Na}) are reduced below their normal levels. Varying the duration of the conditioning pulse reveals that this depression, or *inactivation*, of the g_{Na} takes several milliseconds to develop to its full extent i.e. like the rise in g_K, it is a "delayed" effect of depolarization.

It is clear from this that E_m exerts two opposing effects on the sodium channels: depolarization initiates a rapid opening (activation) and a slow closure (inactivation) of the channels. Thus, the period of high g_{Na} is curtailed by an inactivation process.

The intensity of the inactivation at any given time was found to depend on the strength of the conditioning depolarization—the greater the depolarization, the greater the subsequent inactivation.

One explanation put forward for these findings is that each Na-channel is guarded by two quite separate gates, both of which must be open, at least in part, for the Na ions to penetrate. According to this theory, the two gates in each channel contrast in the speed with which they operate and also in the nature of their response to depolarization: the "fast" Na-gates *open* progressively with depolarization whilst the "slow" Na-gates *close*. Thus, prolonged clamps would initiate a rapid opening of the "fast" gates along with a more leisurely closure of the "slow" gates, and hence account for the transient nature of the rise in g_{Na}. Clearly, the "fast" gates would be responsible for Na-activation and the "slow" gates for the Na-inactivation. (From the time course of the changes in g_K, the K-channels seem to be guarded by single "slow" gates only.)

It will be realized that the magnitude of any transient rise in g_{Na} (due to opening of the "fast" gates) is limited by the state of the "slow" gates. If the "slow" gates are only partly open then they will restrict the passage of ions whatever the state of the "fast" gates. This will be true during voltage clamps and also

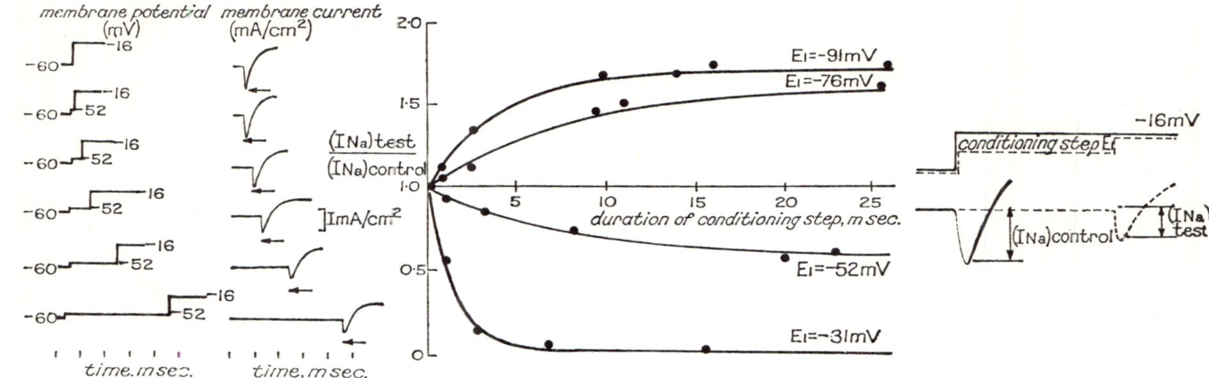

FIG. 50. Inactivation of the sodium channels by prolonged depolarization (squid axon). Recordings: The top trace shows the normal transient sodium current which accompanies depolarizing clamps (control). In subsequent traces, the depolarizing (test) clamp is preceded by a small conditioning depolarization of varying duration. Note the progressive reduction in the initial sodium current as the duration of the conditioning step increases. (The arrows indicate the amplitude of the control current.) Clearly, prolonged depolarization closes up the Na channels: *inactivation*. Graph: Development of inactivation at four different membrane potentials. The ordinate shows the magnitude of the sodium current (test) relative to the normal sodium current (control), measured as indicated in the inset. Note that prolonged depolarization raises the level of inactivation whilst hyperpolarization reduces it and that these effects take a comparatively long time to develop. Thus, the setting of the "slow" gates which are responsible for this inactivation will reflect the steady-state membrane potential. (After Hodgkin & Huxley, 1952c.)

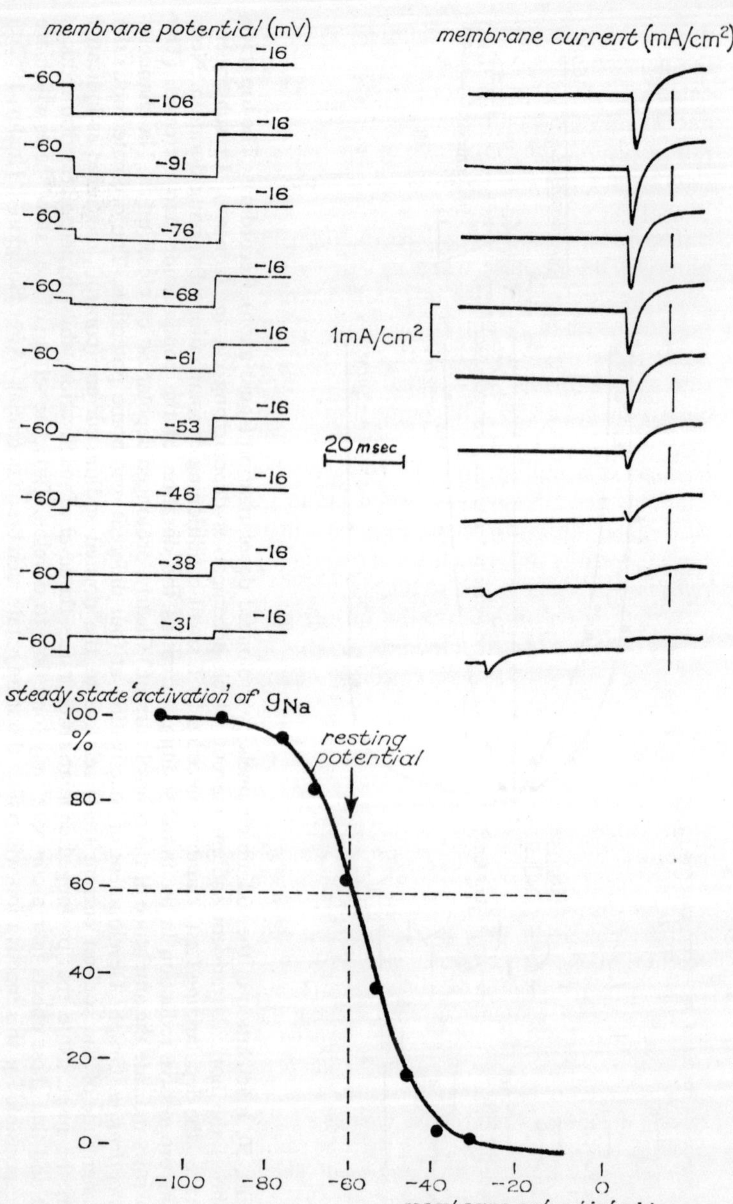
membrane potential (mV)
membrane current (mA/cm²)
-60
-106
-91
-76
-68
-61
-53
-46
-38
-31
-16
1mA/cm²
20 msec
steady state 'activation' of g_{Na}
100
%
80
60
40
20
0
resting potential
-100
-80
-60
-40
-20
0
membrane potential, mV

during impulses in the unclamped axon i.e. it will affect the size of the nerve impulse. At the normal resting potential, these "slow" gates are only 60 per cent open (the axon is 40 per cent inactivated) and even very small changes in E_m could reset them and thus raise or lower the amplitude of the nerve impulse. The functional significance of this will be discussed later in the section on "synapses".

The inactivation of g_{Na} is an important factor in the falling phase of the impulse when its "delayed" effects on g_{Na} coincide with the "delayed" rise in g_K. The combined effects of a fall in g_{Na} and a rise in g_K curtail the main spike and speed the return of E_m to its resting level close to E_K. However, this rapid repolarization will be further accelerated by the direct effect of the potential change on g_{Na} and g_K. In clamped axons, repolarization during the period of high g_{Na} causes a rapid decay in the Na-current in a fraction of a millisecond due to closure of the fast gates in those channels not already inactivated i.e. in those channels where the slow gates are still open. Repolarization during the period of high g_K results in a much slower decay, the K-currents extending over two or three milliseconds.

With a mass of data on the properties of the nerve membrane now at their disposal, Hodgkin & Huxley were able to compute the time course of the permeability changes which follow activation of the unclamped nerve. From this they derived a mathematical description of the nerve impulse which "generated"

FIG. 51. The influence of membrane potential on g_{Na}-inactivation in the steady-state (squid axon). Above: Standard depolarizing (test) clamps are preceded by conditioning pulses of standard duration (sufficient to allow inactivation to reach an appropriate steady-state level) and variable magnitude. Since the amplitude of the sodium current during the test pulse will vary as g_{Na}-inactivation varies, it can be used to reveal the dependence of the "slow" Na gates on membrane potential. (The vertical bars at the side of each current trace indicate the amplitude of the control sodium current.) Below: The graph summarises the nature of this relationship, indicating the level of g_{Na}-activation by plotting the test sodium current as a percentage of the maximum sodium current. Note that the curve is steepest in the region of the resting potential (when the Na channels are less than 60% activated—or 40% inactivated) indicating that the sodium channels in the resting fibre are very sensitive to even small fluctuations in the membrane potential. (After Hodgkin & Huxley, 1952c.)

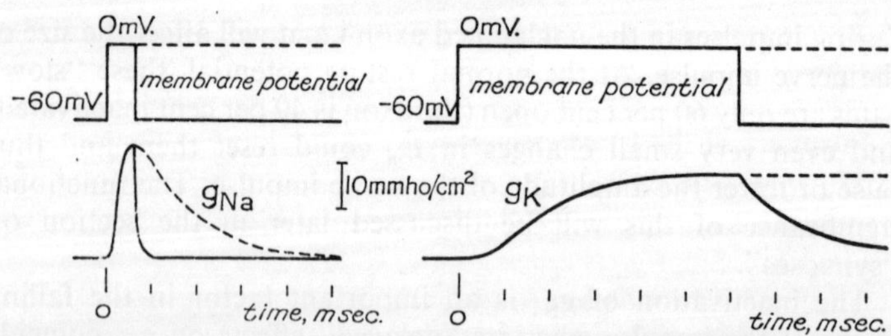

FIG. 52. The effect of rapid repolarization of the membrane during the periods of high g_{Na} and high g_K in the squid axon. Note that on repolarization the decay in g_{Na} proceeds very rapidly (taking a fraction of a millisecond) whilst the decay in g_K is much more leisurely (taking several milliseconds), reflecting the voltage dependence of "fast" and "slow" gates respectively. The broken curves show the characteristic responses to maintained depolarizations. (After Hodgkin, 1958.)

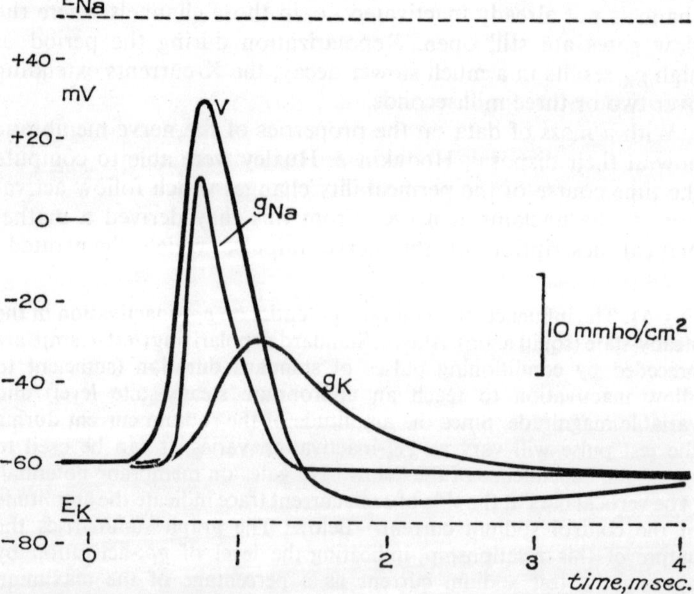

FIG. 53. A theoretical reconstruction of the action potential and conductance changes based upon a numerical analysis of the data derived from the voltage clamp experiments on the squid axon. The calculated exchange of Na and K ions is slightly in excess of 4 picomoles per sq.cm. of membrane. (Hodgkin & Huxley, 1952d.)

spikes displaying a remarkably close resemblance to the recorded variety.

A Summary of the Events which make up the Nerve Impulse

The Rising Phase. Initially, the quiescent membrane is depolarized by the local circuit currents in the vanguard of the approaching impulse. Since g_K is much greater than g_{Na} in the resting nerve, small depolarizations fail to generate spikes because the K-efflux exceeds the Na-influx and so returns the membrane potential to its resting level. It is only when the membrane is depolarized by some 15 mV that the Na-gates open to a sufficient extent for the Na-gain to exceed the K-loss. Once this critical point is reached, Na ions move into the axon under a considerable electrochemical gradient and depolarize the membrane further. The dependence of g_{Na} on membrane potential operates to accelerate the reversal of E_m: depolarization opens the "fast" Na-gates, which thus allows more Na ions to enter the axon, producing further depolarization, etc. This self-reinforcing Na-influx generates the very steep rising phase of the impulse. Once this positive feedback cycle is initiated, the remaining events take a stereotyped form and produce the *all-or-none* impulse.

The Transition Period. As E_m rapidly moves towards E_{Na}, several factors interact to stem the flow of Na ions into the axon and encourage the loss of more K ions. The "delayed" effects of depolarization—closure of the "slow" Na-gates (Na-inactivation) and opening of the K-gates—begin to curb the "runaway" rise in g_{Na} and elevate g_K. Coupled with this is a progressive fall in the electrochemical gradient on the Na ions (as E_m approaches E_{Na}) whilst that on the K ions rises (as E_m moves away from E_K). Thus, the K-efflux increases and eventually exceeds the declining Na-influx. At this point, the membrane starts to repolarize.

Repolarization. As the "delayed" effects of depolarization become firmly established, the transition from a membrane with a high g_{Na} to one with a high g_K proceeds rapidly. With a large driving force on the K ions and only a small one on the Na ions, the brisk loss of K ions quickly repolarizes the membrane. This process is accelerated by a further reduction in g_{Na} which is a direct consequence of the repolarization—the "fast" Na-gates now close and cut off those channels not already inactivated.

The After-Potential. The membrane is now discriminating heavily in favour of the K ions, whose loss drives the membrane towards E_K. During the few milliseconds that it takes for the g_K to return to its resting level and for the reopening or reactivation of the "slow" Na-gates, the membrane is hyperpolarized.

The Recovery. Gradually the resting membrane potential is restored, and the small quantities of Na and K ions which have exchanged between the axon and its surroundings will be made good by the pump.

CHAPTER 4

The Input Signal

Our main concern in this chapter is with the agencies through which the CNS collects information: the receptors. It is the function of each receptor to signal the approach or presence of a particular physical stimulus, and a wide range of sense organs are to be found scattered about the periphery which are selectively sensitive to heat, light, mechanical and chemical agents. By the deployment of an extensive system of such sensors, the brain is able to sample the condition of its environment.

Since the nerve impulse is the only kind of input signal directly acceptable to the brain, the receptors must perform a transducer function, transforming the energy from the external disturbance into analogous neuronal activity. Thus, irrespective of the class of stimulus which activates them, all receptors respond by generating impulses in the afferent fibres which then convey them into the CNS. It is the central connexions of these fibres which alone determines the quality of the sensations evoked by the input message. It is implicit in such a system where each receptor responds preferentially to only one form of energy that the afferent pathways should convey this information separately to appropriate integrating centres in the CNS.

The Receptor Discharge

The receptors encountered in man and animals take a wide variety of forms, some of which are more readily accessible to investigation than others. One receptor, located in the muscle of the abdominal segments of the crayfish, has proved particularly useful because it is large enough to admit microelectrodes for recording purposes (most others have very fine terminals which are much too small to penetrate). Most sense organs seem to share the same basic mechanisms of receptor function and the crayfish stretch receptor—which will be the chief one considered here—can therefore serve as an introduction to receptor mechanisms in general.

When a suitable stimulus is applied to a receptor, it initiates a burst of nerve impulses in the afferent fibre. Fig. 54 shows one such discharge, recorded from the axon of a crayfish stretch receptor in

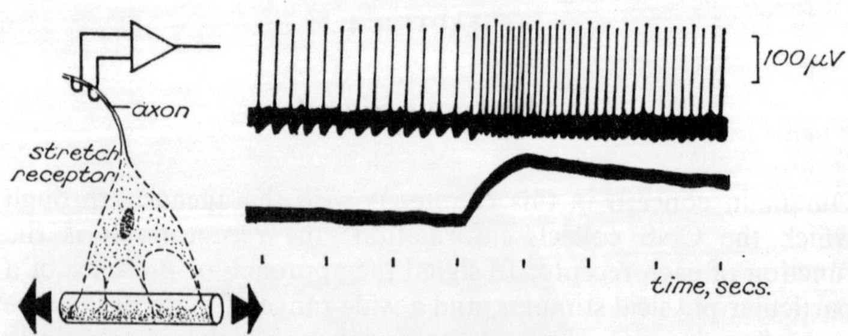

FIG. 54. The discharge from a crayfish muscle stretch receptor in response to an applied stretch. Upper trace: action potentials (note extracellular recording). Lower trace: tension in the muscle. (After Krnjević & van Gelder, 1961.)

response to a light pull on the muscle. Increasing the intensity of the stimulus by further stretch promptly raises the frequency of the discharge. Indeed, the repetition rate of this impulse traffic closely follows the rise and fall of the stretch. The receptor thus provides the CNS with input signals whose frequency correlates closely with the intensity of the applied stimulus i.e. the information is conveyed in the form of a frequency code. The exact, mathematical relationship between stimulus intensity and impulse frequency is difficult to define since it is not clear whether the receptor monitors the magnitude of the applied force or the extent of the resultant stretch (or both). Terzuolo & Washizu (1962) found that the firing rate in the crayfish stretch receptor axon is linearly related to the length of the muscle but varies as the logarithm of the applied force. Investigations on other receptors suggest that the logarithmic function is more usual.

The Generator Potential

It was seen in the last chapter that depolarization is an essential precursor for the rise in g_{Na} which marks the conversion of the membrane to an active state. It follows from this that the receptor mechanism must at some stage depolarize the membrane beyond its firing level in order to initiate nervous activity. Intracellular recordings, made by penetrating the receptor cell with a micropipette, reveal that a steady depolarization always accompanies the stimulus but only fires the cell if it succeeds in reaching a certain critical level (indicated by an arrow in Fig. 55). In all of the

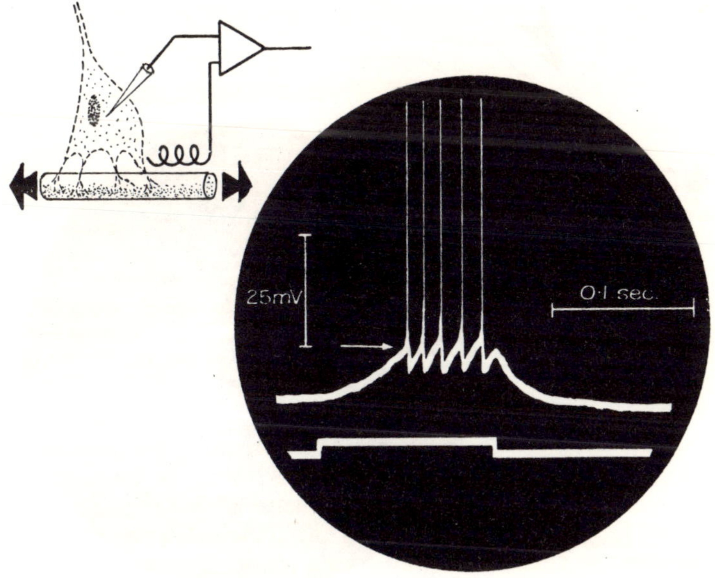

FIG. 55. The receptor discharge from a crayfish stretch receptor recorded with an intracellular microeletrode. Upper trace: action potentials. Lower trace: tension in the muscle. Note the maintained depolarization which accompanies the stretch and which initiates a spike when membrane potential exceeds some threshold (indicated by the arrow). (After Eyzaguirre & Kuffler, 1955.)

sense organs so far investigated, receptor discharges have always been associated with depolarizations, which are now termed *generator* or *receptor potentials.* Clearly, the inference to be drawn from this is that the generator potential represents an essential part of the receptor mechanism and is directly concerned with setting up the afferent impulses.

The drug, cocaine, has been widely used in investigations into receptor mechanisms since it blocks the regenerative processes which are necessary to support impulses but has little effect on the generator potential. Under these circumstances, the generator potential can be studied in isolation and is not obscured by the impulses. Such recordings underline the sharp contrast between

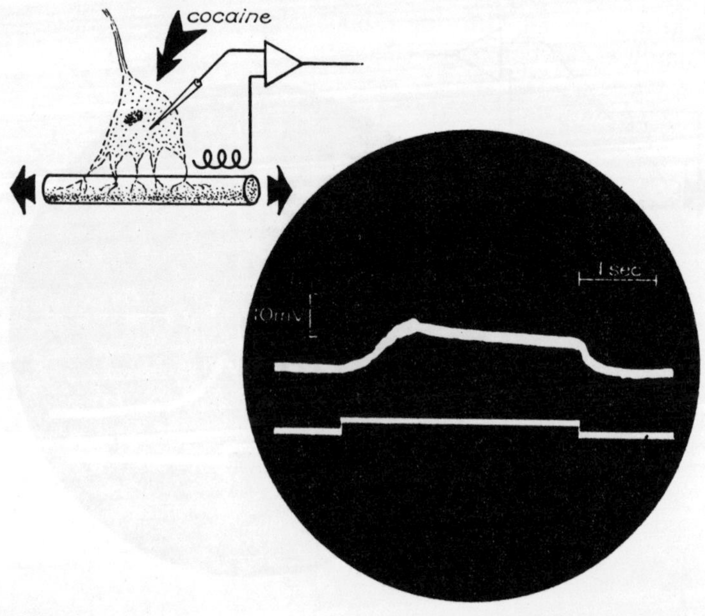

FIG. 56. An intracellular recording from the crayfish stretch receptor showing the generator potential which accompanies an applied stretch. Upper trace: membrane potential. Lower trace: tension in the muscle. Spike activity has been abolished by prior treatment with cocaine. (After Eyzaguirre & Kuffler, 1955.)

propagating, all-or-none nerve impulses and the strictly local, continuously-graded, generator potentials. Thus, the generator potentials can only be recorded in the immediate vicinity of the receptor and their magnitude varies with the intensity of the stimulus (c.f. the electrotonic potentials).

The above investigations suggest that the generator potential is an intermediate stage in the transduction processes at the receptor and that its only function is to initiate the receptor discharge in the afferent fibre. The overall transformation, stimulus—generator potential—spike discharge, is a logarithmic function, and since the firing rate in the axon varies directly with the amplitude of the generator potential, the logarithmic relationship must reflect the transducer function per se (Fig. 57).

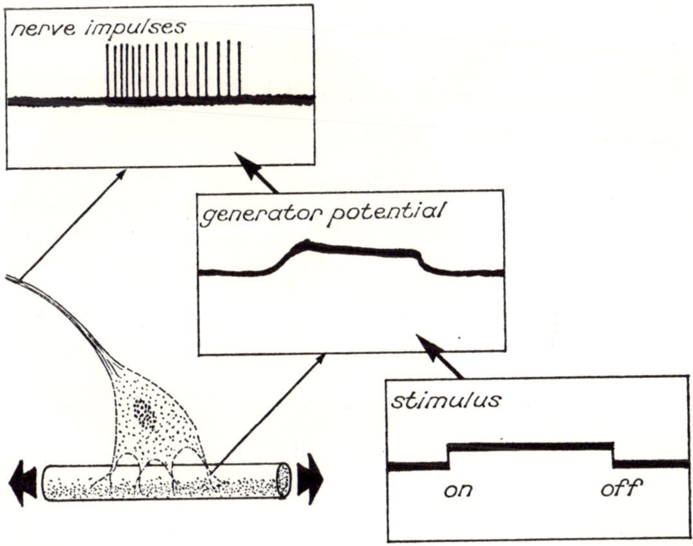

FIG. 57. A summary diagram showing stages in the genesis of the receptor discharge. The receptor produces a local potential profile of the stimulus—the graded generator potential—which in turn triggers propagating, all-or-none impulses in the axon.

Origin of the Generator Potential

Having suggested that the generator potential plays a central role in the production of a nervous discharge which is appropriate to the applied stimulus, we shall now focus our attention on the genesis of this potential. Terzuolo & Washizu (1962) observed a significant rise in the conductance of the receptor membrane during stretch of the crayfish muscle and suggested that this was responsible for the local depolarization. These workers impaled the receptor with two micropipettes, one being used to manipulate the membrane potential whilst the other recorded the effect of this on the amplitude of the stretch-induced generator potential. If the latter results from stretch-induced permeability changes, then altering E_m would be expected to change the driving forces on

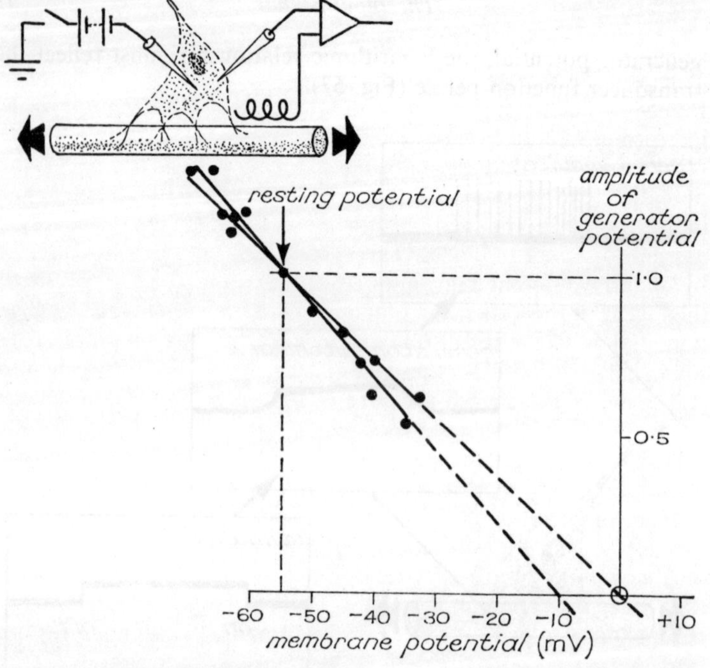

FIG. 58. The equilibrium potential for the generator currents at the crayfish stretch receptor. If the generator potential arises from permeability changes and is due to ions moving down their electrochemical gradients toward their equilibrium potential, then shifting the membrane potential towards this equilibrium potential should reduce the amplitude of the generator potential and vice versa. Because this stretch receptor is unusually large, it has been possible to introduce a pair of microelectrodes into it, one to pass current (and hence shift membrane potential to some new level) whilst the other records the generator potentials resulting from standard stretches. Unfortunately, this technique only permits manipulation of membrane potential over a small range, but extrapolation indicates that the generator potential would reverse at some value between 0 mV and − 10 mV—the equilibrium potential for the generator currents. One further difficulty with this technique is that the manipulation and recording are done at the cell body whilst the channels carrying the generator currents are probably some distance away in the dendrites. It could well be that the current passed from the microelectrode has less effect on the transmembrane potential in the region of these channels than the recording electrode suggests so that the "true" curve is somewhat steeper than the one shown. (After Terzuolo & Washizu, 1962.)

the ions involved and so modify the amplitude of the subsequent generator potential. The results are summarised by the graph in Fig. 58, which shows that the generator potential was raised by an increase in E_m and lowered by a decrease. Extrapolation of these results suggests that the currents associated with the generator potential tend to drive E_m towards zero (approximately), hence indicating that the equilibrium potential for the "generator currents" is close to 0 mV. (This same conclusion can be deduced by slightly different reasoning. If the extrapolation is justified, then clearly, the generator potential reduces with the membrane potential and reverses at 0 mV. Thus, if E_m could be reduced by some means to 0 mV, subsequent stretch of the muscle would still open up the stretch-sensitive channels in the receptor membrane, but the net "generator currents" would be zero i.e. the ions carrying the "generator currents" would be equilibrated. 0 mV must therefore represent the equilibrium potential for the "generator currents".)

Since no single ion has an equilibrium potential near 0 mV, we must conclude that the "generator currents" are carried by more than one ion. The simplest view—which is still in need of experimental verification—is that the generator potential results from a non-selective increase in membrane permeability. This would imply that the membrane simply "perforates" and allows all ions (i.e. Na, K and Cl ions) to flow along their electrochemical gradients, thereby discharging the membrane. In the absence of further data, it is unwise to pursue the mechanism in more detail.

It is apparent from the intracellular records shown above that the receptor membrane is able to support both spike activity and the generator potential simultaneously. We can assume therefore, that the stretch-sensitive channels are comparatively few in number and hence insufficient to "short-out" the spike.

The existence of relatively few stretch-sensitive channels would also explain why the generator potential rarely exceeds 20 mV even with maximal stretch, when the "theoretical" limit is nearer 60 mV. Of course, the actual number of channels opened up will vary with the degree of stretch and so give rise to continuously-graded depolarizations. However, any shift in membrane potential away from the resting level uncovers driving forces which augment the resting "leakage" currents and tend to restore the resting potential. Thus, these resting "leakage"

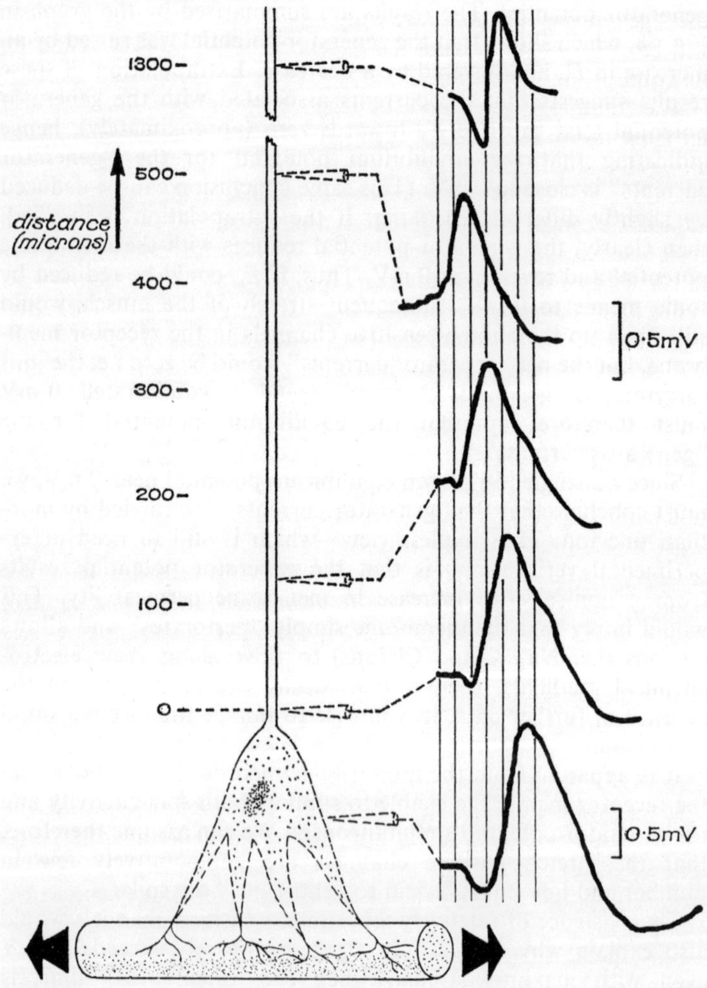

FIG. 59. The origin of the nerve impulses in the lobster muscle stretch receptor. With one electrode inside the cell body and the other placed at various points along the axon, it is clear that the earliest spikes following stretch arise some 500 microns along the axon. Thus, the spikes recorded at the cell body have originated in the axon—where

channels will tend to short-circuit the generator potential. Since the "generator currents" are only small, the "leakage" currents will be sufficient to prevent the generator potential ever achieving its equilibrium condition.

The impulses generated by the receptor are not actually initiated in the body of the receptor cell, but arise some distance along the axon. Edwards & Ottoson (1958) recorded the receptor discharge at various points along the length of the cell body and adjacent axon of the lobster stretch receptor and found that the conducted spikes first appear some 500 microns away from the cell body (see Fig. 59). However, the permeability changes—and hence the "generator currents"—which result directly from the stretch are probably restricted to the fine receptor endings so that the generator potential spreads into the adjacent cell body and axon through the action of local circuit currents. These local exchange currents will encounter considerable longitudinal resistance in the axon and the associated generator potential will attenuate severely with distance. Since the axon fires *before* the cell body inspite of this decrement in the generator potential, it must be assumed that the threshold for self-reinforcing impulses is lowest in the axon. Nonetheless, spikes are recorded from the body of the receptor and it is now clear that these impulses have "back-fired" into the cell body from the axon. Thus, the impulses which make up the receptor discharge are initiated in the first part of the axon and propagate in both directions away from this area, i.e. into the CNS, and into the receptor cell body.

Coding of the Input Message

It would be a gross error to consider the receptor input to our brain as a complete and faithful analogue of the environment; this it certainly is not. Firstly, our receptors are highly selective and only sample some of the physical characteristics of the world around us. Secondly, of the information that our receptors do supply, much of it is a severely abbreviated and even distorted version of the original input. This is merely to admit that there is a

---

presumably the threshold is very low—and only secondarily invade the cell body. The vertical lines provide a time scale, representing intervals of 0·1 msec. Note that the recordings are extracellular and that the lowest trace has been obtained at a lower gain than the rest. (After Edwards & Ottoson, 1958.)

limit to the brain's capacity to assimilate incoming signals, and evolution has resulted in our dependence on selected inputs only.

In the remainder of this chapter, we shall enquire into the range and fidelity of the information which receptors make available to the CNS. For this purpose, the brain can be regarded as an immense information processing system whose input resources are limited to the five senses. Each receptor can be regarded as a pass filter, transmitting information concerning one specific parameter in the environment and rejecting all others. Thus, although our eyes are very sensitive to electromagnetic waves ranging in wavelength from 4 to 7 millimicrons, they are completely unresponsive to the much longer radio waves. Similarly, the human ear does not embrace the high-frequency "sounds" emitted by the bat's sonar system. It is only through modern technology that man has been able to extend his cognisance of the physical world beyond the constraints of the five senses.

If a stimulus is so delicate that the resulting generator potential fails to depolarize the afferent fibre to threshold, then the CNS will not be made aware of the existence of that stimulus. Clearly, it is desireable that receptors should be as sensitive as possible, and certainly, some of our sense organs are exquisitely responsive. Individual receptors in our eyes can detect the presence of a single quantum of light, whilst some sounds are discernible even when they deflect the eardrum by as little as the width of a hydrogen atom!

However, at the other end of the intensity scale, all receptors show *saturation*. When the intensity of the stimulus exceeds a certain maximum, further increases in its magnitude will evoke no further response from the receptor. The sense organ is said to be saturated and generates impulses at its maximum frequency, which may be several hundred per second. Thus, each sensory unit embraces the whole of its monitoring range in a frequency code extending from zero to a few hundred impulses per second. When it is realized that the eye, for instance, is responsive to luminance changes over a range of about 10^{10}, it is clear that individual receptors could not possibly monitor the whole range except with the grossest sensitivity. This raises a difficulty which is common to all recording systems: how to retain high sensitivity to small changes in the input and, at the same time, cover a wide range? The nervous system tackles this problem in a number of ways which reveal some important features about our sensory system:

1. *Parallel Structuring of Sensory Systems.* In any population of receptors of a similar type e.g. the stretch-sensitive ones in muscle, there will be a wide range of thresholds and saturation levels. This will mean that as the intensity of the stimulus increases, units of progressively higher and higher thresholds will be recruited. Thus, as some sensory units are approaching saturation others will be coming up to their thresholds, thereby extending the monitoring range beyond that of the individual receptor.

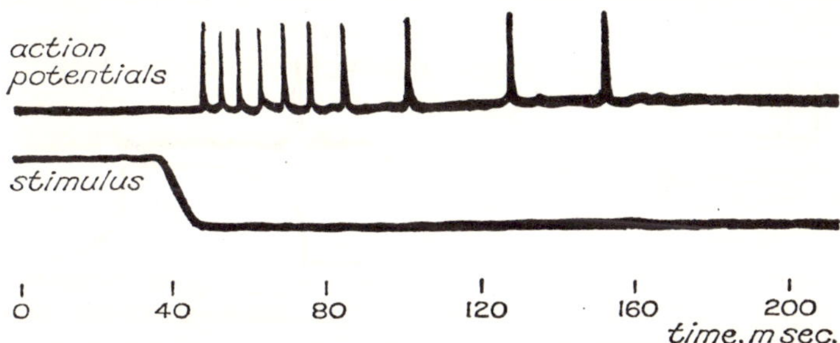

FIG. 60. The receptor discharge from a rapidly adapting touch receptor in the toad. Upper trace: action potentials (extracellular). Lower trace: stimulus. Note the rapid decay in the firing rate even though the stimulus is maintained: *adaptation.* (After Lindblom, 1962.)

2. *Adaptation.* Many receptors do not respond to steady, maintained inputs with continuous discharges, but merely generate bursts of impulses at the "on" and "off". Such receptors are only sensitive to *changes* in the stimulus and so provide information which is differentiated with respect to time. An extreme example of this type is the pacinian corpuscle, which is found in the skin, mesentery, tendons and joints of mammals where it responds to mechanical distortions. When a steady, maintained pressure is applied to this receptor, it rarely produces more than one spike and then falls silent until the pressure is either released or increased. The rapid fall in the firing rate even though the stimulus is maintained is called *adaptation.*

All receptors show some adaptation and are distinguished on the basis of the *rate* at which they adapt to the input. Slowly adapting receptors such as the crayfish stretch receptor, are often called "tonic" receptors and tend to maintain their firing levels during steady stimuli. Rapidly adapting receptors like the pacinian corpuscle are said to be "phasic" because they only respond to the rise and fall of the input.

Loewenstein & Mendelson (1965) showed that the phasic properties of the pacinian corpuscle are imparted by the viscoelastic nature of its investing lamellae. Thus, when the lamellae were carefully stripped away and the stimulus applied directly to the exposed nerve terminal, the rate of adaptation was considerably reduced. Using flash microphotography, Hubbard (1958) showed

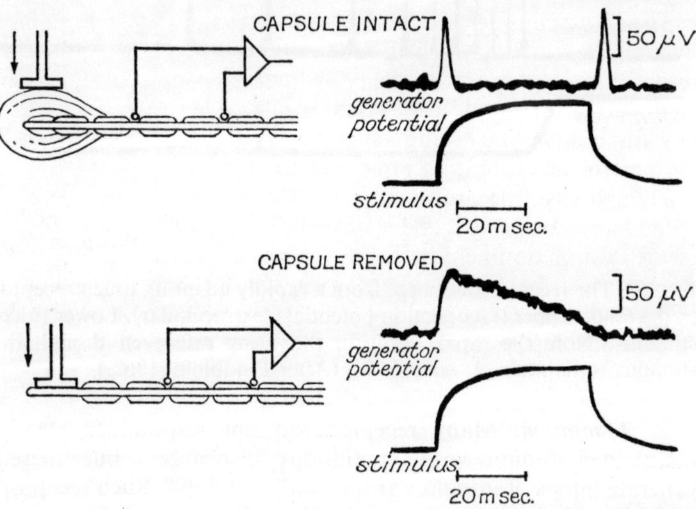

FIG. 61. Adaptation at the Pacinian corpuscle of the cat. Upper traces: the normal generator potential recorded with the capsule intact. Note the very rapid adaptation with only transient ON-OFF responses. Lower traces: the generator potential after removal of the capsule. Note the much slower decay of the ON response and the complete absence of an OFF response. Throughout these recordings, the preparation was treated with cocaine, thereby abolishing any action potentials which might have obscured the generator potentials. (After Loewenstein & Mendelson, 1965.)

that the lamellae oppose rapid distortion i.e. they possess considerable viscous friction, and so transmit the full force of transient stimuli to the central nerve terminals. When the stimulus is maintained, the lamellae balloon out to accommodate it and hence distortion of the terminals is curtailed. The time course of the generator potential thus correlates with the distortion of the nerve terminals.

In general, rapidly adapting receptors will keep the animal informed on the "new" developments in the environment and at other times remain quiescent. These input signals are ambiguous, in that they fail to distinguish between the "on" and the "off" of the stimulus, and taken individually, also fail to give any indication of the "absolute" intensity of the stimulus. However, they do succeed in maintaining a very high sensitivity over a wide range of input levels.

The above considerations might suggest that, in achieving a high dynamic sensitivity which is wide ranging, the rapidly adapting receptor has had to trade fidelity and hence produces only a poor analogue of the input. This would surely be a very high price to pay for a wider recording range unless there were other good reasons for incorporating rapid adaptation into the system.

Though vast, the processing capacity of the nervous system is by no means unlimited, and is obviously incapable of handling all of the information held by the environment. This means that the system must be highly selective in the information which it chooses to process, operating stringent economies to keep the volume of receptor traffic within manageable proportions and also to achieve optimum utilization of its resources. The nervous system has therefore concentrated its monitoring resources on those features of the environment which are of particular survival value. Judged in this light, much of the information in the surroundings is irrelevent.

Rapidly adapting receptors reflect this need to "optimize the useful" in responding preferentially to *change* in the environment and ignoring the static, background levels. Clearly, information on the moving features in the vicinity will be of immense survival value since both food and predators will enter this category at an early stage in their influence. Our own nervous system seems to be particularly sensitive to dynamic stimuli in a number of different ways; we can perceive moving objects in the periphery of our visual field much more readily than stationary ones, and rapid temperature or pressure changes much more readily than slow ones. These effects are not due entirely to adaptation at the receptor level and in part reflect central processes, but they serve to emphasize how our nervous system has optimized reception of dynamic features. The static features are predictable after a

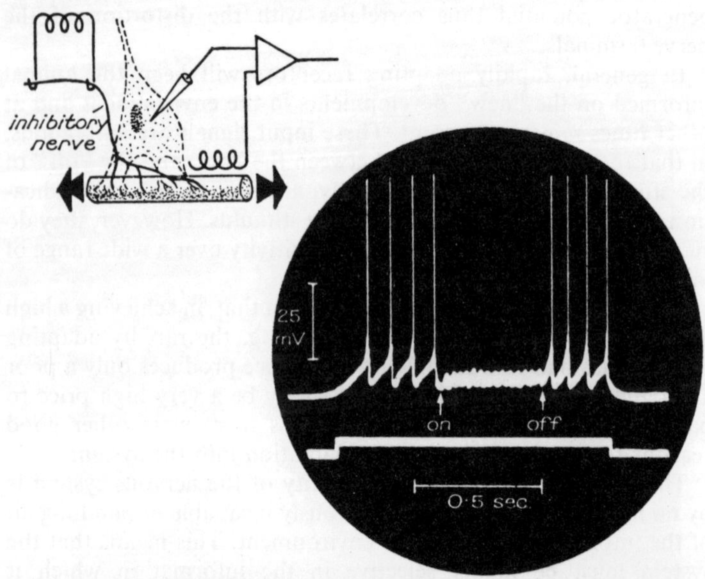

FIG. 62. Inhibition at the crayfish muscle stretch receptor. Upper trace: action potentials recorded with an intracellular electrode. Lower trace: tension in the muscle. When the inhibitory axon is stimulated at 34 per second (between the arrows) there is a partial repolarization of the membrane and consequently a complete arrest of the receptor discharge. Thus, the inhibitory input has the effect of switching the receptor off and rendering it less sensitive to stretch. (After Kuffler & Eyzaguirre, 1955.)

FIG. 63. The equilibrium potential for the inhibitory currents at the crayfish muscle stretch receptor (E_{inh}). The inhibitory input to the receptor acts through a chemical transmitter substance which attenuates the generator potential by modifying the permeability of the receptor membrane. Stimulation of the inhibitory axon leads to a shift in membrane potential towards E_{inh}, and in the normal resting condition the inhibitory potentials are depolarizing (trace C, each inhibitory volley being indicated by an arrow). When the membrane potential is reduced by prior stretch of the muscle, i.e. using the generator potential to adjust E_m to new levels, the inhibitory potentials become strongly polarizing. The graph summarizes these findings and reveals that the inhibitory input always drives E_m towards − 55 mV (E_{inh}). (After Kuffler & Eyzaguirre, 1955.)

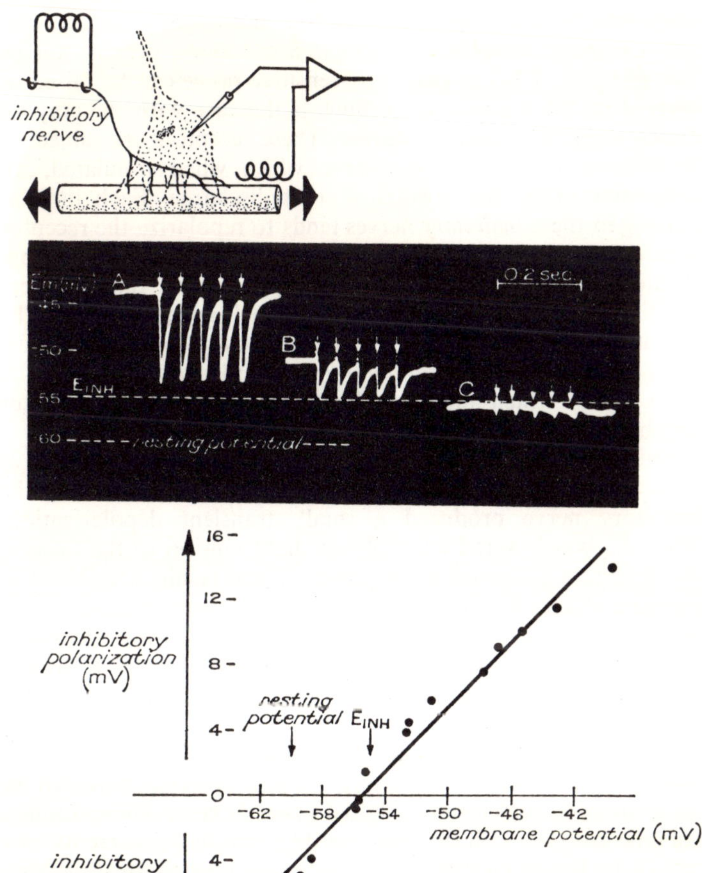
inhibitory
nerve
Em(mV) A
0·2 sec.
-45
-50
B
EINH
55
C
60 resting potential
16
12
inhibitory
polarization
(mV)
8
resting
potential
EINH
4
0
-62
-58
-54
-50
-46
-42
membrane potential (mV)
inhibitory
depolarization
(mV)
4
8

preliminary assessment, and provided that they remain so, are not worthy of further scrutiny by the nervous system. The tedious repetition involved in continuous monitoring of unchanging features can obviously be very wasteful of computer time and space and should be kept to a minimum.

3. *Central Control of Receptors.* Some sense organs can be "reset" by the CNS so that their sensitive range can be raised or lowered to the required level. Such is the case with the crayfish stretch receptor considered earlier. These receptors are subject to the influence of certain motor nerves which, when stimulated, can completely arrest the normal afferent discharge. Each impulse arriving in these *inhibitory* nerves tends to repolarize the receptor membrane and thereby oppose the stretch-induced depolarization. In effect, this switches the receptor on to a new "range" where the discharge rates for each level of stretch are now lower. The inhibitory nerves bring about these effects by releasing a chemical agent (probably gamma-aminobutyric acid: Hagiwara, Kusano & Saito, 1960) which modifies the permeability of the receptor membrane.

Kuffler & Eyzaguirre (1955) found that when E_m was at its normal resting value—about -60 mV—stimulation of the inhibitory nerve produced a small, transient depolarization. When E_m was lowered by applying slight tension to the muscle, the inhibitory potential was reversed. These results are shown in Fig. 63 and it is clear from the graph that the reversal potential for the inhibitory currents was about -55 mV. Edwards & Hagiwara (1959) found that when K ions were removed from the bathing solution, there was the expected rise in E_m but, in addition, the inhibitory potentials became more strongly hyperpolarizing. Hagiwara *et al.*, (1960) exchanged the external Cl ions for glutamate and found little change in E_m whilst the reversal potential for the inhibitory currents was shifted towards zero. These findings are all consistent with the view that the "inhibitory currents" are carried by K and Cl ions. E_{Na} is so far removed from the inhibitory reversal potential that Na ions are unlikely to be involved.

The inhibitory influence tends to oppose the normal stretch-induced depolarization by stabilizing E_m near its resting level and thereby preventing any shift towards threshold. Thus, the firing rate in the afferent fibre will be determined by the balance between the central repolarizing influence and the stretch-induced depolarization, so that in effect, the receptor is "biassed" by the inhibitory impulse traffic. A similar resetting mechanism is found in the vertebrate muscle stretch receptor and has attracted considerable attention from the control engineers who have applied the mathematical concepts used in servo-engineering in an attempt to explain their significance. However, this raises problems outside the province of this book.

CHAPTER 5

The Synapse

The information processing carried out in the CNS involves the transfer of signals across intricate networks of neurones. In the course of this data handling, fresh information is introduced into the system from the receptors and is sorted, weighed against other factors and ultimately shaped into some pattern of activity which will provide appropriate action. Sophisticated processing of this kind requires an immensely elaborate organization, and structurally, the system is a profusion of interconnexions which defies formal description.

The function of the neurone in this, is to provide an integrating surface where signals can be brought together, sifted and fashioned into an output signal. The axon, of course, provides for the immediate dispatch of this output signal to the next integrating centre. Thus, the individual unit functions like a nervous system in miniature.

The extensive stretch of membrane investing the body of the neurone and its projecting dendrites—the soma-dendritic membrane—composes the receiving area for the whole cell, and is covered with the swollen end-feet of hundreds or even thousands of axon terminals which deliver the input signals for processing. A narrow gap separates each of these axon terminals from the underlying membrane and presents such a high resistance to the local circuit currents associated with the incoming spikes that they fail to invade it. Transmission across these junctions, or synapses, is therefore discontinuous, and the functional link between neurones is provided by chemical transmitter processes. These involve a chemical transmitter substance which is stored in the presynaptic axon terminal and is released into the gap on the arrival of an impulse. Diffusion then carries the transmitter on to the postsynaptic membrane. The effect of this transmitter agent on the postsynaptic membrane varies from synapse to synapse, and there appear to be a variety of such substances released by different terminals. However, all of these chemical agents seem to bring about their effects on the target neurone by modifying the permeability of its membrane. We have seen that permeability changes can have a profound influence on the membrane potential

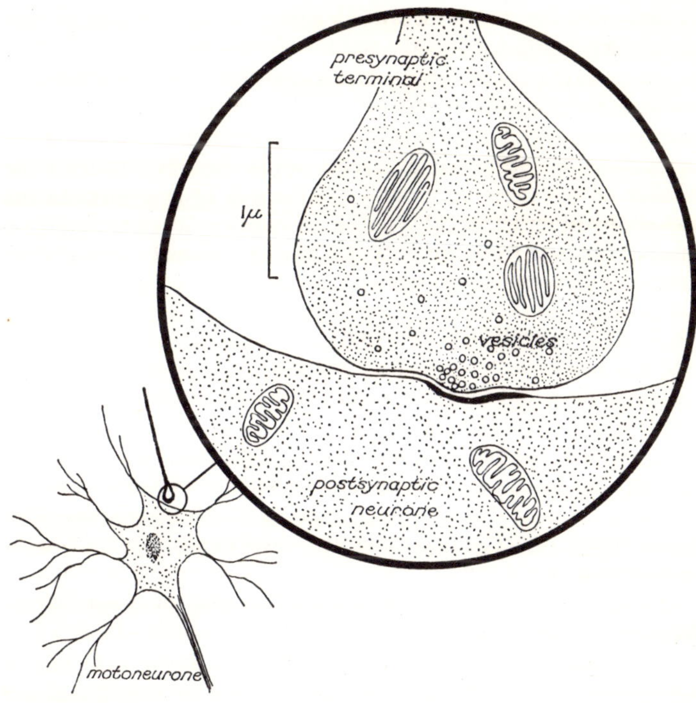

FIG. 64. A diagram of a neuronal synapse based upon electron micrographs.

and, in general, either depolarize the cell towards its firing level, or stabilize the membrane at some level below threshold and hence oppose any tendency for the cell to fire. It is therefore not surprising to find that impulse traffic in some presynaptic fibres tends to augment the activity of the postsynaptic neurone (excitation) whilst signals arriving at other endings tend to depress it (inhibition).

The activity of each neurone is governed by the balance between these excitatory and inhibitory inputs. However, the large number of inputs involved, coupled with the complex geometry of the cell body and its dendrites, present the investigator with formidable problems when he tries to study these integrative processes. Our first concern here is with the mechanics of synaptic transmission i.e. the processes leading to the release of the transmitter substance and the nature of its subsequent action on the postsynaptic membrane. For this purpose, it is convenient to consider a synapse at which no integration occurs and which is readily accessible: the vertebrate neuromuscular junction. It seems that the sequence of events which occurs during transmission across these peripheral junctions is little different from that at any other chemical synapse, so that we can draw freely on much of the data from these studies when we come to consider the more complex central synapses.

The Frog Neuromuscular Junction

It is usual in vertebrates for each muscle fibre to receive only one nerve fibre and for the nerve-muscle junction to function as a simple slave relay: every nerve impulse which arrives at the junction, or *motor end-plate* as it is called, generates a corresponding impulse in the muscle fibre. When these two impulses are recorded together it can be seen that an interval separates them which cannot be accounted for entirely by transmission time in the nerve terminal and muscle fibre. This delay between the arrival of the presynaptic spike at the nerve terminals and the generation of the postsynaptic spike in the muscle fibre is usually about 0·5 to 0·8 msec. The sequence of events contributing towards this delay is common to all chemical synapses and must include:

1. Mobilisation of the transmitter substance stored in the presynaptic nerve terminals.
2. Presynaptic release of the transmitter into the synaptic cleft.
3. Diffusion of the transmitter across the cleft and on to the postsynaptic membrane (in this particular case, the muscle).
4. Reaction time between transmitter and hypothetical receptor molecules at special sites on the postsynaptic membrane.
5. The opening up of ionic channels in the postsynaptic

FIG. 65. The ultrastructure of the frog neuromuscular junction. Above: an impression of the general relationship between the motor nerve terminal and muscle fibre. Below: a tracing from an electron micrograph of a longitudinal section through the junction. The arrows indicate the basement membrane which partitions the gap between the nerve and muscle and provides a core for the postsynaptic folds. (The calibration bar is only approximate.) (After Birks, Huxley & Katz, 1960.)

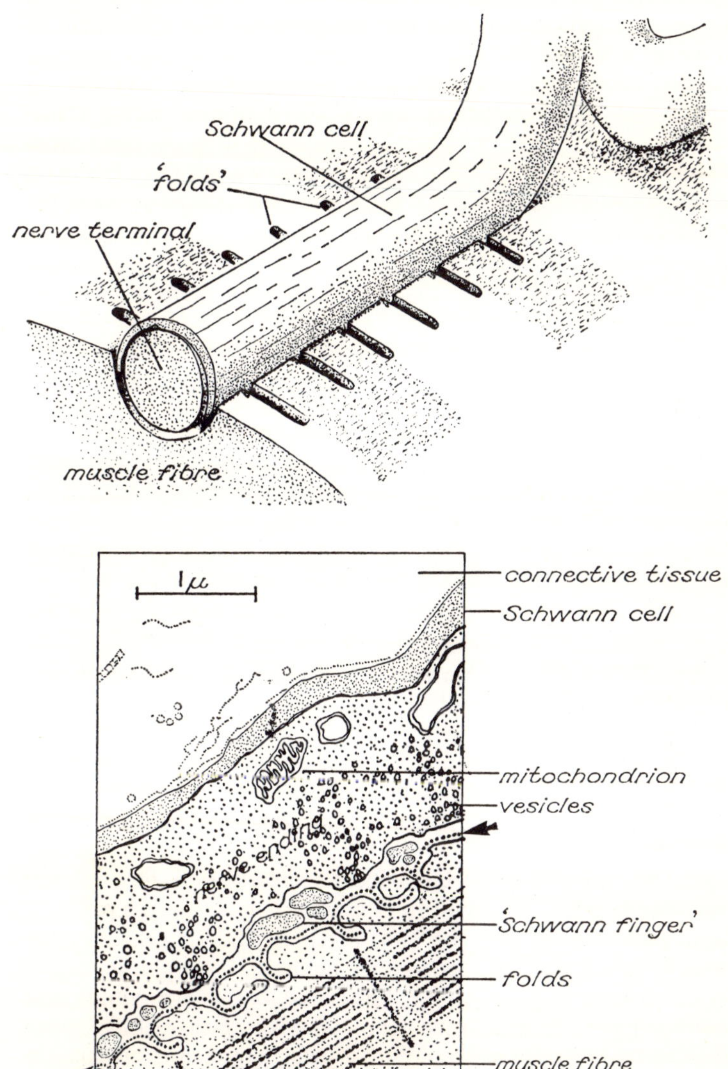
Schwann cell
'folds'
nerve terminal
muscle fibre
1μ
connective tissue
Schwann cell
mitochondrion
vesicles
nerve ending
'Schwann finger'
folds
muscle fibre

membrane. (In this particular case, this results in depolarization of the muscle to threshold and hence sets up a propagating impulse there.)

In the early 1930's several workers had suspected for some time that the transmitter substance was acetylcholine (ACh), but attempts to detect it in the perfusate draining the junction had proved unsuccessful. It was later found that there were other substances present at the synapse which hydrolyse the ACh (the cholinesterases), and it was only after these had been inactivated with so-called anti-cholinesterases (such as eserine), that detectable quantities of ACh escaped into the perfusate (Dale, Feldberg & Vogt, 1936). The quantity of ACh collected correlates very closely with the frequency of the impulses arriving in the presynaptic nerves and Krnjević & Mitchell (1961) estimate that each impulse promotes the release of several million molecules of ACh at each end-plate.

The direct application of ACh to the nerve-muscle preparation can give rise to normal muscle spikes and hence, contraction. However, minute quantities of ACh administered through a micropipette are only effective in the immediate vicinity of the end-plate and much larger quantities are required to evoke spikes from regions only a millimeter or two away (del Castillo & Katz, 1955). Clearly, the muscle membrane at the end-plate is a very sensitive ACh-detector.

The Effect of the Transmitter Substance on the Postsynaptic Membrane. When the muscle impulse is recorded with an intracellular micropipette in the region of the motor end-plate, it has a slightly distorted form compared with similar records taken from more remote areas of the muscle, and amongst other things, shows an inflexion in the rising phase. This inflexion becomes more apparent when the drug, curare, is applied to the preparation and represents the leading edge of a local depolarization, *the end-plate potential* (e.p.p.). Under normal circumstances, the e.p.p. depolarizes the muscle fibre beyond threshold and so generates the muscle impulse (c.f. the generator potential.). If the concentration of the curare is raised, the e.p.p. is reduced in magnitude and eventually fails to depolarize the muscle fibre to threshold. Under these conditions, there is a failure in neuromuscular transmission in so far as no muscle impulse is generated and hence no contraction develops, although small e.p.p.'s can still be recorded. Further increases in the drug level lead to the total suppression of

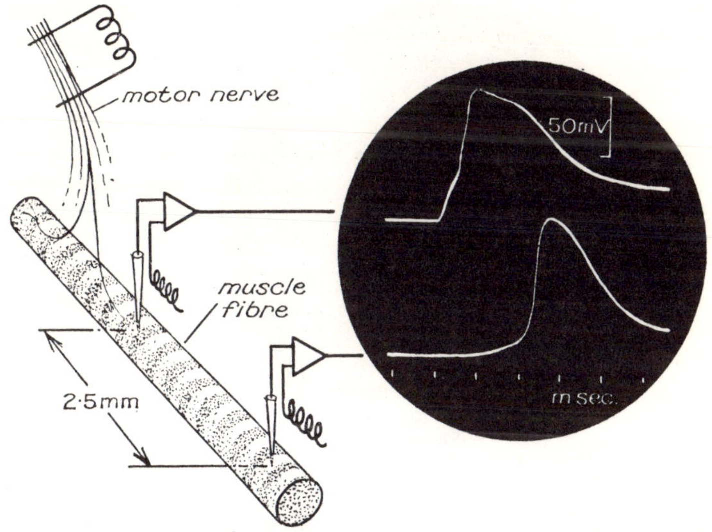

FIG. 66. Action potentials recorded from a frog muscle fibre with intracellular micropipettes in the end-plate region (upper trace) and the periphery (lower trace) in response to a single volley in the motor nerve. Note the "irregularities" in the form of the end-plate spike. (Fatt & Katz, 1951.)

the e.p.p. Since the usual quantities of ACh can still be collected from these curarized preparations (Dale *et al.*, 1936), it is clear that the drug does not interfere with the release of the transmitter and must be acting postsynaptically. However, the drug does not impair the muscle's capacity for conducting impulses since these can still be evoked by direct electrical stimulation of the muscle. The curare must therefore block neuromuscular transmission by rendering the postsynaptic membrane less responsive to ACh, probably by commandeering the essential "receptor" sites.

Intracellular recordings in the muscle fibre disclose that the e.p.p. attenuates rapidly with distance and is restricted to the region of the end-plate (Fatt & Katz, 1951). This establishes that the e.p.p. is a local depolarization resulting from local transmitter action at the end-plate and must be clearly distinguished from the propagating impulse which it initiates. Furukawa,

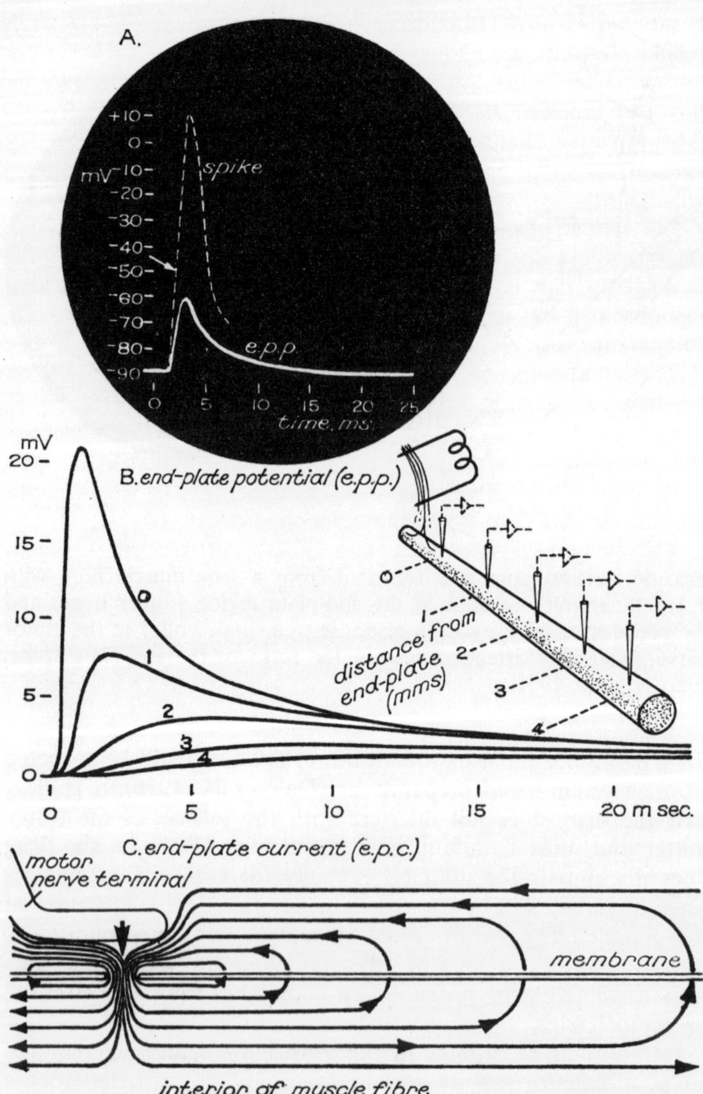

FIG. 67. The end-plate potential at the frog neuromuscular junction. A: an intracellular recording from the end-plate region of the muscle showing the response to a single volley in the motor nerve after treat-

Sasaoka & Hosoya (1959) have shown that TTX, which selectively blocks Na-channels, abolishes all impulse activity in the nerve and muscle, but spares the local depolarization which follows the direct application of ACh to the junction. This suggests that the ACh-sensitive channels which carry the end-plate currents and generate the e.p.p. are quite separate from the Na-channels which carry the action currents.

The failure of the e.p.p. to spread much beyond the end-plate region is usually of no significance since the e.p.p. normally depolarizes the muscle fibre beyond threshold and the local response matures into a self-reinforcing impulse which travels the full extent of the fibre.

These experiments reveal that the normal muscle spike is triggered by a local, non-propagated depolarization, the e.p.p., which arises from the action of ACh on the muscle membrane at the end-plate. It is now firmly established that the ACh exerts these effects by increasing the permeability of the postsynaptic membrane. Let us examine this evidence more closely:

The membrane potential of the resting muscle fibre is usually about −90 mV and is reversed during the impulse, which may have an amplitude of up to 125 mV. Careful analysis of the form of the muscle spike reveals some consistent distortions in recordings made in the region of the end-plate, in addition to the inflexion in the rising phase which has already been mentioned.

---

ment with curare. This drug reduces the effectiveness of the transmitter substance and results in a failure of transmission at the synapse. However, in suppressing the spike, a local synaptic response, the end-plate potential (e.p.p.), is revealed, albeit in a slightly reduced form. It is this e.p.p. which under normal circumstances is sufficiently large to depolarize the membrane beyond threshold (indicated by the arrow) and initiate the propagating muscle spike which activates the contractile mechanism. B: the form of the e.p.p. when recorded at various distances away from the end-plate with an intracellular electrode (figures on each trace indicate the distance, in millimetres, from the end-plate). Note the decremental propagation, the e.p.p. becoming progressively smaller and slower towards the periphery of the muscle. C: the end-plate currents (e.p.c.) responsible for the generation of the e.p.p. Transmitter action opens up channels in the muscle membrane at the end-plate which allow sufficient flow of current to discharge the membrane capacitance and depolarize the muscle fibre beyond threshold. (After Fatt & Katz, 1951.)

Thus, the amplitude of the spike is usually reduced by about 15 mV whilst the falling phase is interrupted by a "hump" which delays the repolarization of the membrane (see Fig. 66).

Fatt & Katz (1951) suggested that these irregularities were due to local permeability changes following transmitter action in the end-plate region i.e. the ACh opens up channels in the membrane which remain open after the initiation of the spike and so in part short-circuit the normal action currents. In order to be quite certain that these distortions were due to transmitter action and were not due to differences in the properties of the membrane at the two recording sites, Fatt & Katz recorded muscle impulses from the end-plate region which were produced (*a*) by the

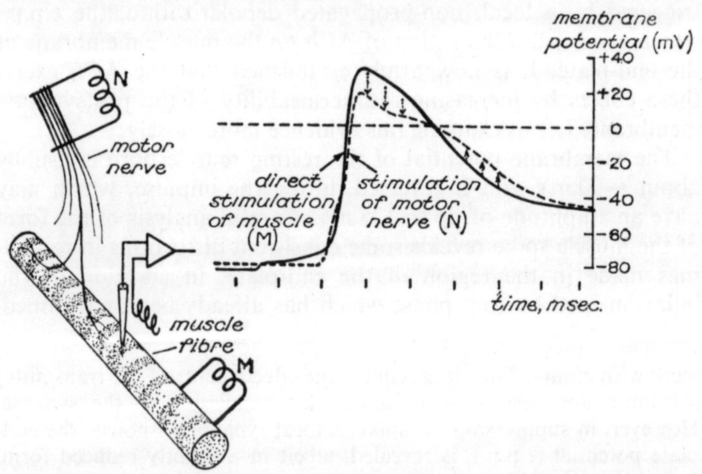

FIG. 68. Intracellular recordings of muscle action potentials in the end-plate region of frog muscle. The continuous line shows the response following direct electrical stimulation of the muscle (at M), when the impulse is merely picked up as it passes through the end-plate region. This response is hardly different from that normally recorded in the periphery of the muscle. The discontinuous line is the normal trans-synaptic response recorded from the end-plate, i.e. in response to motor nerve stimulation (at N). In both of these recordings, action currents successfully generate a spike, but it is clear that the presence of transmitter substance modifies the membrane in such a way as to reduce the peak of the spike and slow its decay, i.e. it tends to stabilize E_m at some value near zero (approximately). (After Fatt & Katz, 1951.)

normal synaptic processes following motor nerve stimulation, and (*b*) by direct electrical stimulation of the muscle (see Fig. 68).

The muscle spikes evoked by direct electrical stimulation of the muscle were found to be little different from those normally observed in the periphery of the muscle, indicating that the distortions in the normal end-plate spike must originate from transmitter action. Furthermore, the irregularities were always such as to shift membrane potential towards 0 mV. This plainly suggests an approximate value for the reversal potential of the end-plate current (E_{epp}). In an attempt to obtain a more accurate value for E_{epp}, del Castillo & Katz (1954) used a very ingenious "collision technique" which involved the stimulation of both the motor nerve and the muscle fibre together, so that the end-plate membrane was invaded simultaneously by the ACh from the motor nerve terminal and the antidromic spike*. In this way, the antidromic spike was used to alter membrane potential during the period of transmitter activity and thus provide a variable driving force for the ions generating the e.p.p. By varying the interval between the two pulses, it was possible to arrange for the ACh to arrive at the postsynaptic membrane when the membrane potential was any value from −90 mV (the resting potential) up to +35 mV (the peak of the antidromic spike). Fig. 69 illustrates some of the results obtained in this study and shows how the E_{epp} averaged about −15 mV, a value subsequently confirmed by voltage clamp techniques (Takeuki & Takeuki, 1959). These voltage clamp experiments were later repeated in solutions of different ionic compositions in an attempt to identify the ions carrying the end-plate current (Takeuki & Takeuki, 1960). Removing cations (Na or K ions) from the external solution increased the E_{epp} whilst alterations in $[Cl]_o$ had no effect. This suggests that ACh renders the postsynaptic membrane permeable to Na and K ions only,† which seems reasonable since E_{epp} (−15 mV) falls in between the values of E_{Na} (about +50 mV) and E_K (probably about −100 mV).

*Although nerve and muscle fibres can transmit impulses in either direction along their lengths, they are normally only called upon to carry information in one direction—the *ortho*dromic direction. It is possible to set up impulses which proceed in the reverse, or *anti*dromic, direction by direct electrical stimulation of the nerve or muscle.

†In postulating channels which are permeable to cations only, it is necessary to explain how the "large" Na ions can penetrate whilst the "small" Cl ions are excluded. One suggestion is that the channels contain fixed negative charges which repel all anions and thereby prevent them from gaining access to such channels.

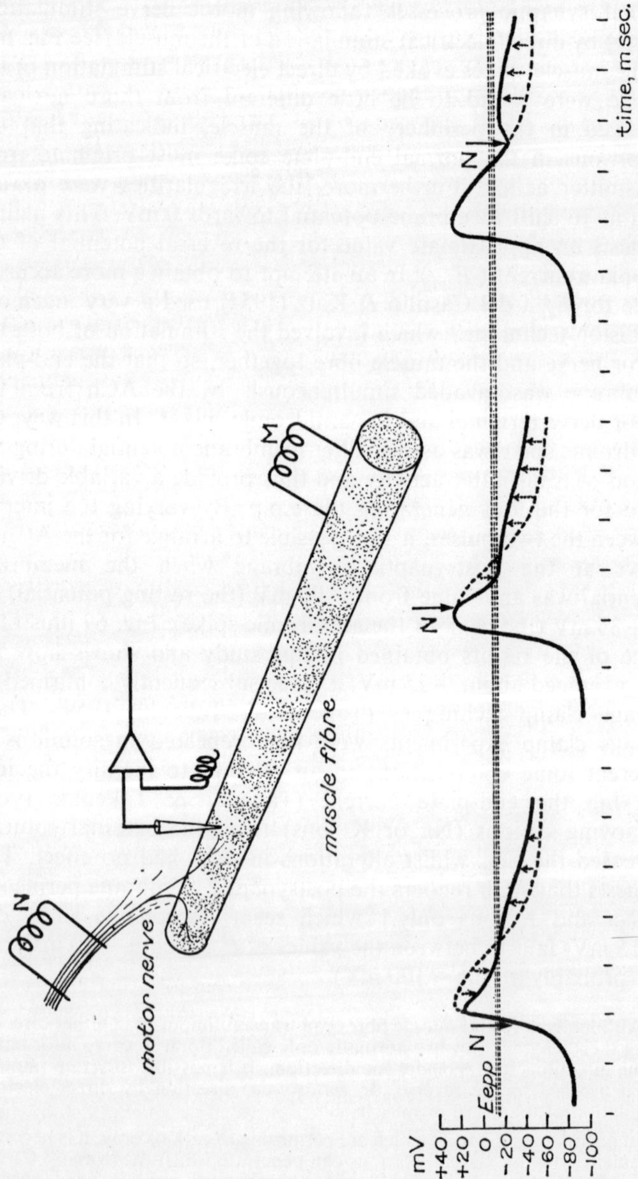
N
motor nerve
muscle fibre
M
mV
+40
+20
0
−20
−40
−60
−80
−100
Epp
time, m sec.

The Quantal Nature of the Transmitter Release. Recently there has been considerable interest in the mechanisms which lead to the release of the transmitter substance by the axon terminals. Much of this originates from a chance observation made by Fatt & Katz whilst they were engaged upon intracellular recordings in the end-plate region of frog muscle fibre (Fatt & Katz, 1950, and reported more fully, 1952). These workers observed small, spontaneous depolarizations (usually about 0·5 mV) which seemed to occur at irregular intervals in the absence of any impulse activity in either the nerve or muscle. Since these potentials were suppressed by curare and enhanced by anti-cholinesterases, it was clear that they resulted from the action of ACh on the postsynaptic membrane. At first it was thought that they were simply due to leakage of ACh from damaged nerve terminals, but it later became apparent that they were genuine biological phenomena and were not artefacts. A remarkable feature of these miniature potentials was their uniformity of size in any given muscle fibre, suggesting that they represent the effect of discrete packets of ACh rather than some periodic molecular overspill.

From a functional point of view, these miniature potentials can only be regarded as low-level synaptic "noise", their amplitudes being only about 1 per cent of the normal e.p.p. and far too small to depolarize the muscle to firing level. However, Fatt & Katz succeeded in demonstrating a relationship between these miniature potentials and the e.p.p. which has subsequently

---

FIG. 69. Intracellular recordings of muscle action potentials in the end-plate region of frog muscle (the "collision technique"). In these experiments, direct electrical stimulation of the muscle (at M) is closely followed by a stimulus to the motor nerve (at N) timed to bring about transmitter release as the spike due to the first stimulus is traversing through the end-plate region. Clearly, if transmitter action modifies the permeability of the postsynaptic membrane (muscle), then it would be expected to distort any spike coursing through the end-plate. The arrows (labelled N) indicate the approximate time at which the transmitter action commences. The waveform of the "undistorted" muscle spike set up by stimulation at M has been traced in (discontinuous line) to emphasize the nature of the effects. It is clear that the transmitter-sensitive channels tend to stabilize E_m at approximately $-$ 15mV (E_{epp}). (After del Castillo & Katz, 1954.)

proved to be of immense significance. They pointed out that, like e.p.p.'s, these miniature depolarizations could only be recorded from the muscle membrane immediately beneath the motor nerve terminals and were never recorded from any area which failed to yield e.p.p.'s. Except for their low amplitude and the fact that they occurred spontaneously, the miniature potentials resembled the normal e.p.p. so closely that Fatt & Katz called them *miniature e.p.p.'s* and suggested that they constituted the basic, or quantal, unit of transmitter action. The e.p.p. was therefore assumed to result from the synchronous release of many small packets of ACh, each of which individually would produce a miniature e.p.p.

These ideas have since been examined in more detail and it has proved particularly useful to study the system in calcium-deficient solutions. It has long been known that Ca ions are essential for the release of ACh and that removing Ca ions from the external solution leads to a block in neuromuscular transmission (Cowan, 1940). Fatt & Katz found that reducing the external Ca ion levels had little effect on the miniature potentials but produced a profound reduction in the amplitude of the e.p.p. Furthermore, in the later stages, this reduction occurred in a stepwise fashion. This last observation accords exactly with the quantal theory of transmitter release, which predicts that the amplitude of the e.p.p. should reduce through a series of "preferred" amplitudes corresponding to the number of quanta released.* The reduction in the e.p.p. only becomes "stepwise" when the response reaches very low levels, i.e. the statistical composition of the e.p.p. is only readily discernible when a small number of quanta are involved. At other times, the e.p.p. is made up of so many units that all evidence of its quantal structure is lost in the summation.

A number of workers have since applied rigorous statistical analysis to the reduced e.p.p.'s found in low-calcium solutions and have firmly established the validity of the quantal theory (del Castillo & Katz, 1954a; Boyd & Martin, 1956; Liley, 1956; Katz & Miledi, 1965c). In the experiments of Boyd & Martin on the cat neuromuscular junction, the spontaneously occurring miniature e.p.p.'s had a mean amplitude of 0·4 mV. Solutions deficient in

*Such a series could only be obtained through an effect on the *number* of quanta released and in the absence of any effect on the *size* of the individual quanta. The fact that the size of the miniature e.p.p. is unaffected by low-calcium solutions is consistent with its postulated quantal role.

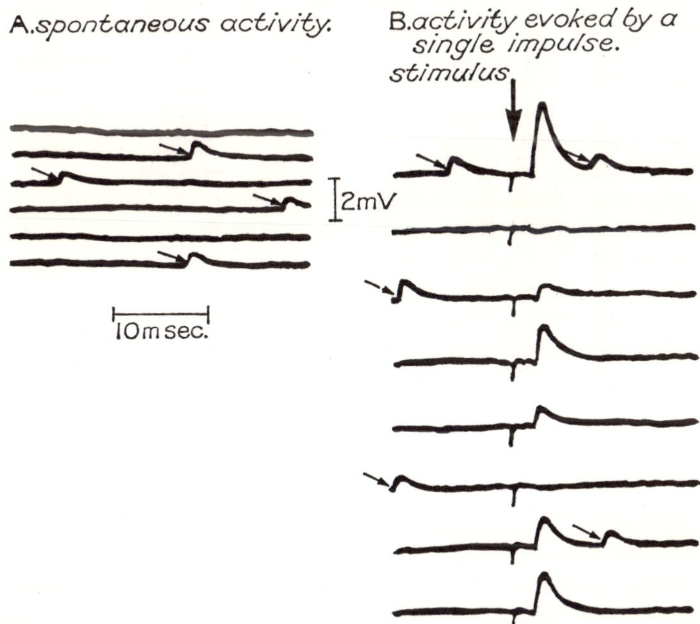

FIG. 70. Intracellular recordings from the end-plate region of rat diaphragm. A: spontaneous activity in the form of miniature potentials, each indicated by an arrow. B: the e.p.p. resulting from single volleys in the motor nerve in Ca-deficient and Mg-rich solutions. Such solutions effectively restrict the transmitter release to a few, readily discernible quanta, hence the large "quantal" fluctuations in the amplitude of successive e.p.p.'s. (After Liley, 1956.)

Ca ions produced large reductions in the e.p.p. evoked by single shocks to the motor nerve and, on average, their amplitudes tended to be simple multiples of the miniature potentials, i.e. 0·4 mV, 0·8 mV, 1·2 mV, 1·6 mV, etc. These regular fluctuations in the magnitude of the ep.p. are clearly due to variations in the quantal content, whilst their consistent relationship with the miniature potentials establishes the latter as the basic unit or *quantum of transmitter action.*

Having proved the "physiological existence" of preformed units of ACh in the presynaptic terminals, it is of interest to

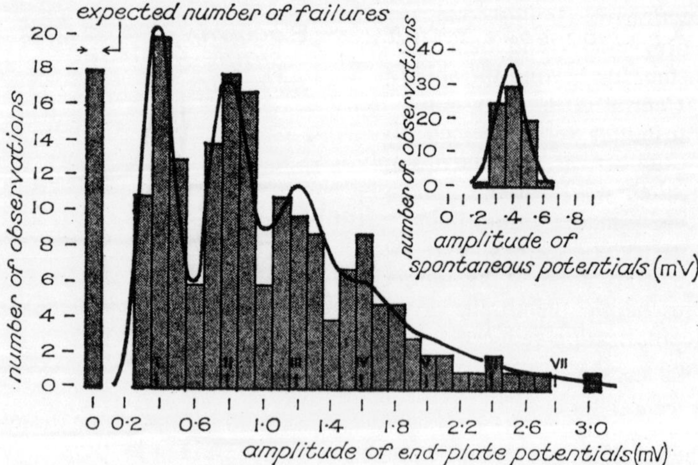

FIG. 71. Amplitude histograms of e.p.p.'s and spontaneous miniature potentials (inset) from cat neuromuscular junction in Mg-rich solutions. The e.p.p. amplitudes are not evenly distributed over the whole range but show peaks at 1, 2, 3 and 4 times the mean amplitude of the spontaneous miniature potentials. A Gaussian curve has been fitted to the miniature potentials and used to calculate the theoretical distribution of e.p.p. amplitudes (indicated by the continuous curve), assuming each e.p.p. to be compounded of one or more miniature potentials. (Boyd & Martin, 1956.)

demonstrate their anatomical existence. For this, we must turn to the electron microscope and it is very encouraging to find that a number of authors describe small vesicles in the presynaptic terminals, approximately 500Å in diameter, which could probably satisfy the physiologist's requirements (Robertson, 1956, 1960; Birks, Huxley & Katz, 1960). There is some evidence which suggests that the ACh in these terminals is concentrated in the vesicles (Whittaker, 1964; de Robertis, 1964), but it still remains to be seen if the vesicles correspond to the preformed units mentioned above. According to this vesicular hypothesis, the miniature potentials found at the quiescent junction result from the all-or-none release of ACh from the individual vesicles overlying the cleft. However, this spontaneous, low frequency activity at the junction seems to have little functional significance, the important event being the arrival of an impulse which, in a fraction of a millisecond, synchronizes the discharge of 150 or more vesicles and hence secures depolarization of the muscle membrane beyond threshold.

Control of the Transmitter Release. It is clear that the normal transmitter release which gives rise to the e.p.p. is triggered by the arrival of a nerve impulse at the presynaptic terminals. In their work on the squid giant synapse, Takeuki & Takeuki (1962) made intracellular recordings from both pre- and postsynaptic fibres and were able to alter the size of the presynaptic spike indirectly by passing current across the presynaptic membrane from a third micropipette: prolonged depolarization reduced the spike size (by increasing the level of the g_{Na}-inactivation) whilst hyperpolarization produced the reverse effect. These experiments showed that the number of quanta of transmitter released—as indicated by the amplitude of the resultant postsynaptic potential—was governed by the size of the presynaptic spike. Thus, an increase of 30 mV in the amplitude of the presynaptic spike produced a 10-fold rise in the postsynaptic potential (see Fig. 72).

It is very pertinent at this juncture to enquire which particular feature of the invading impulse actually triggers the transmitter release: the change in membrane potential, the Na-influx and/or the K-efflux? When the Na-channels in the presynaptic terminals are blocked with TTX, the miniature e.p.p.'s continue unabated and depolarization of the terminals with applied current from a microelectrode can increase their frequency and even produce normal e.p.p.'s (Elmqvist & Feldman, 1965; Bloedel, Gage, Llinas & Quastel, 1966, 1967; Katz & Miledi, 1967b.). Similar results were obtained when the K-channels were blocked with TEA (Katz & Miledi, 1967b). Clearly, the nervous control of secretion is fundamentally an electrical process and is not dependent on the Na and K fluxes which attend the nerve impulse.

In a recent series of experiments, Katz & Miledi (1965a, b & c) sought to obtain more accurate information about the time course of the various events leading up to the production of the e.p.p., and in particular, about the factors responsible for the synaptic delay i.e. the time which elapses between the arrival of the presynaptic spike and the commencement of the e.p.p. Katz & Miledi made the very interesting suggestion that the delay was due in the main to a delay in the actual release mechanism and that all other factors, including the diffusion time across the cleft, were of

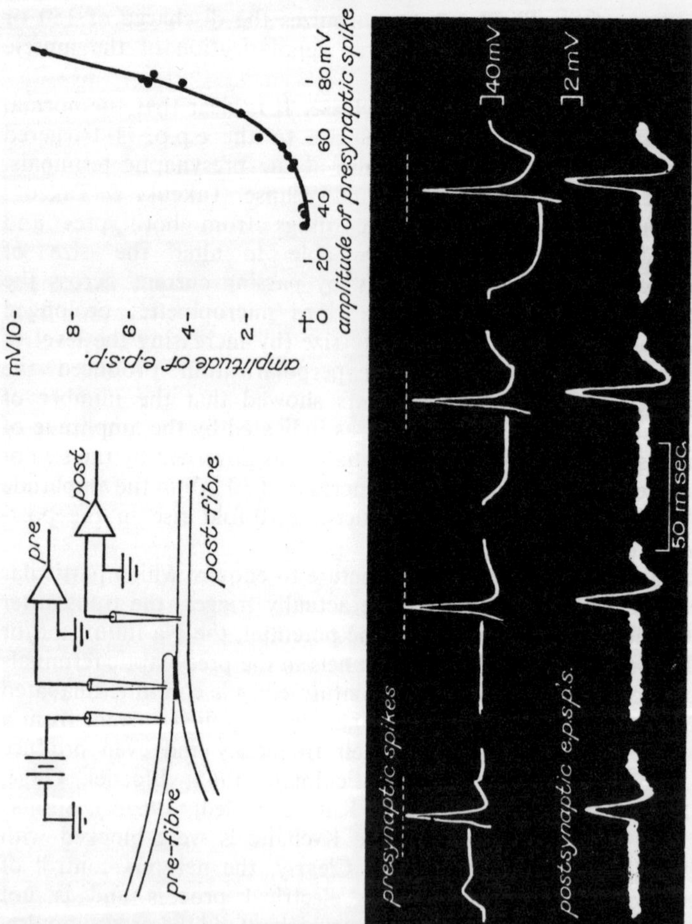

FIG. 72. The dependence of transmitter release on the amplitude of the presynaptic spike at the squid giant synapse. With micropipettes in the pre- and postsynaptic fibres, it is possible to relate the magnitude of the transmitter release (as indicated by the amplitude of the postsynaptic potential, p.s.p.) to the size of the presynaptic spike. The latter was varied in successive experiments by passing current from a second micropipette in the presynaptic terminal. Such currents can produce prolonged changes in membrane potential which raise or lower the level of g_{Na}-inactivation and hence allow manipulation of the action currents and their associated potentials. In the first pair of

minor account. The first experiments were performed at a temperature of 20°C, when the delay had a minimum duration of 0·4 to 0·5 msec., and Katz & Miledi decided to repeat their investigations at a much lower temperature in the hope that the release mechanisms would be slowed down and so permit a closer scrutiny of the sequence of events. Thus, at 2·5°C the total delay was 3·5 to 7·0 msec. In order to obtain some estimate of the diffusion and reaction times, they applied iontophoretic pulses of ACh to the region of the end-plate from a micropipette.* This procedure sometimes depolarized the postsynaptic membrane after a delay of only 0·17 to 0·3 msec., which is less than 10% of the total delay given above. It could be argued that the tip of the micropipette used to administer the ACh was closer to the receptor sites on the postsynaptic membrane than the nerve terminals which normally release the transmitter, hence accounting for this brief latency. However, this seems unlikely, and indeed, one would expect the reverse to be the case i.e. the "true" diffusion and reaction times are likely to be shorter still!

These investigations suggest that the transmitter release is a delayed effect of depolarization (c.f. the rise in g_K and g_{Na}-inactivation during the impulse) and it is interesting in this respect that the release can be suppressed by hyperpolarizing the nerve terminal during the falling phase of the invading impulse (Katz & Miledi, 1967a). What events follow depolarization and are so vital for transmission that the release mechanism awaits them?

*This technique involved passing minute currents from a micropipette loaded with acetylcholine chloride. When the interior of the micropipette is made positive with respect to the surrounding solution, some of the resulting current will be carried out of the tip by the positively charged ACh ions. Thus, voltage pulses can be used for the rapid application of ACh to restricted areas of the end-plate. This technique has a general application for the "injection" or "removal" of ions and has been used extensively to change the concentrations of the various ions inside the cell bodies of central neurones.

---

records, a depolarizing pulse results in slight reductions in the amplitude of both the presynaptic spike and the p.s.p. (as measured against the controls shown in the second pair of records). In subsequent traces, hyperpolarizing pulses increased the amplitude of the presynaptic spike and this resulted in corresponding increases in the p.s.p., indicating augmented transmitter release. The graph summarizes this relationship. Note that although hyperpolarizing pulses increased the amplitude of the presynaptic spikes, the *absolute* potential reached by the peaks was actually reduced. (After Takeuki & Takeuki, 1962.)

Interest at the present time centres around the idea that the initial stages in the release involve an influx of Ca ions. Katz & Miledi (1967c) have found that the Ca ions necessary for the release are only utilized *during* the presynaptic impulse. Transmitter release can be facilitated by iontophoretic pulses of Ca ions which precede depolarization by a mere fraction of a millisecond, but application immediately afterwards is ineffective.

The current view is that depolarization triggers the transmitter release by promoting a delayed rise in the Ca-permeability of the terminal membrane. It is assumed that the Ca ions then enter the nerve terminal under the influence of their electrochemical gradient and must take up essential sites on the inner aspect of the membrane for the transmitter release to proceed. This idea originates, at least in part, from observations made by Hodgkin & Keynes (1957) on the Ca-fluxes in squid giant axons. These workers found that whilst the resting axon is practically impermeable to Ca ions ($P_K : P_{Ca} = 1000 : 1$), nervous activity is associated with an influx of Ca ions, presumably due to a rise in P_{Ca} which accompanies each nerve impulse. However, in order to satisfy the present hypothesis, it is necessary to demonstrate a definite link between this Ca-influx and transmitter release.

In their latest experiments, Katz & Miledi (1967d) have turned to the squid giant synapse, where the presynaptic terminal is large enough to permit intracellular recordings. Their recording arrangements were very similar to those used by Takeuki & Takeuki (1962) with micropipettes in the pre- and postsynaptic fibres for voltage monitoring and a third micropipette to apply depolarizing currents to the presynaptic axon (see Fig. 73).

FIG. 73. Transmitter release at the squid giant synapse induced by strong depolarization of the presynaptic terminal. The disposition of the recording electrodes is the same as in the previous figure. The preparation was treated with TTX and TEA, abolishing all spike activity and making it possible to depolarize the presynaptic terminal by some 200mV or more for prolonged periods; in effect, the terminal membrane is being voltage clamped. Initially, the depolarizing "clamps" produce a delayed ON-release, but as the interior of the terminal is made more and more positive, this is gradually replaced by an OFF-release. The graph shows this transition very clearly, and the complete suppression of the ON-release at potentials above about + 130mV provides an approximate value for the equilibrium potential for the "releasing currents"—E_{RC}. (After Katz & Miledi, 1967d.)

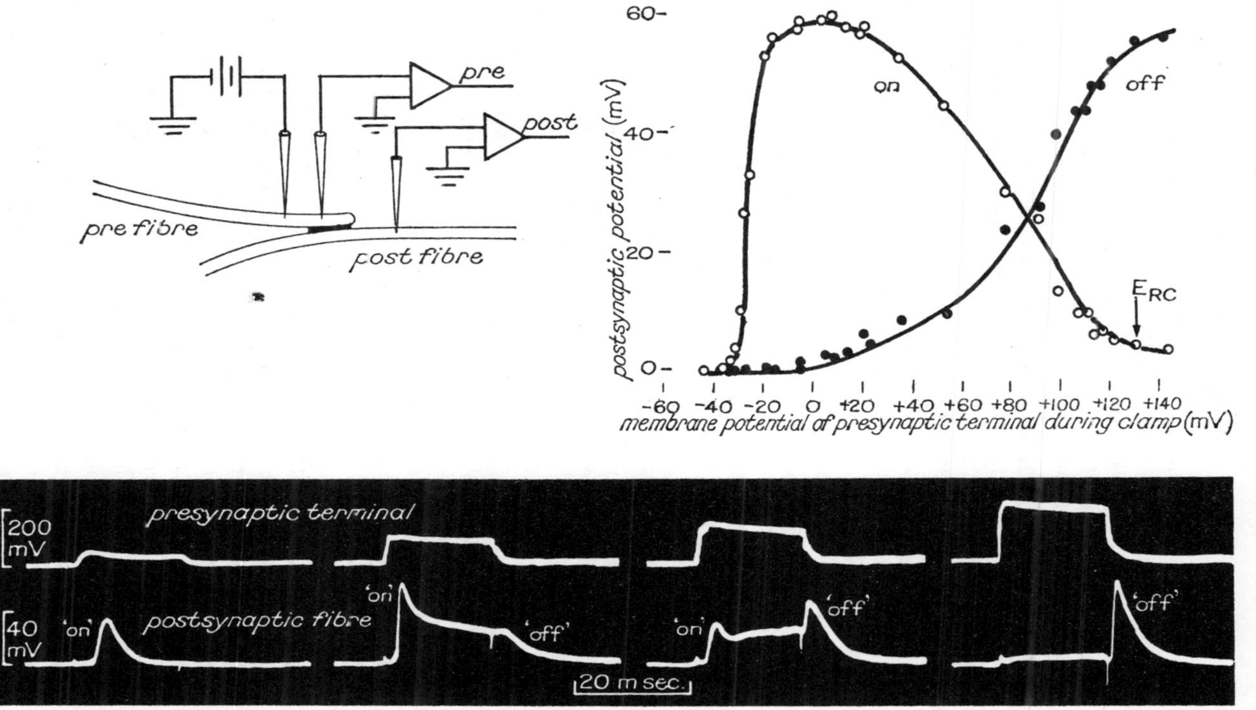
pre
post
pre fibre
post fibre
on
off
E_{RC}
postsynaptic potential (mV)
60
40
20
0
-60 -40 -20 0 +20 +40 +60 +80 +100 +120 +140
membrane potential of presynaptic terminal during clamp (mV)
200 mV
presynaptic terminal
40 mV
'on'
postsynaptic fibre
'on'
'off'
'on'
'off'
'off'
20 m sec.

However, in addition, the presynaptic terminal was loaded with TEA and immersed in TTX so that the K and Na channels were blocked and all impulse activity abolished. With this arrangement, it was found possible to shift the presynaptic membrane potential to any desired level and hold it steady i.e. the presynaptic terminal could be voltage clamped. The experimental procedure involved the depolarization of the presynaptic fibre to some steady voltage whilst monitoring the transmitter release during this time by recording the postsynaptic potential. If depolarization does trigger an inward migration of Ca ions, then clearly the magnitude of this influx will vary with the clamp voltage and will reduce to zero as membrane potential approaches the Ca equilibrium potential (E_{Ca}). The "calcium hypothesis" predicts that transmitter release will fail when the presynaptic E_m reaches E_{Ca} since Ca ions will not enter the terminal and take up the essential "reaction sites". Thus, if the inside of the presynaptic fibre is made sufficiently positive, then transmitter release should be suppressed.

Fig. 73 shows the nature of the transmitter release following the application of various depolarizing clamps to the presynaptic fibre. With weak depolarizations there is a brief postsynaptic potential which follows some three or four milliseconds after the onset of the clamp. With stronger depolarizations, the postsynaptic response increases briskly in both amplitude and duration, soon persisting throughout the full duration of the clamp. However, as successive clamps make the presynaptic potential more and more positive, the postsynaptic potential declines progressively and is replaced by an "off" response.

Transmitter release (as indicated by the size of the postsynaptic potential) is completely suppressed during clamps which raise the presynaptic membrane potential above +130 mV i.e. the equilibrium potential for the essential "releasing currents" (E_{RC}) is about +130 mV. The surge of transmitter release which attends repolarization of the presynaptic fibre can be compared with the surge of current following repolarization during the period of high g_K (p. 58). Thus, it can be explained if we assume that the rise in membrane permeability which promotes the "releasing currents" is maintained throughout the clamp and decays exponentially on repolarization. The residual conductance which temporarily survives repolarization could permit a brief flow of "releasing current" along the new electrochemical gradient and so initiate further transmitter release. The delayed and gradual rise in the transmitter release at the onset of depolarization is consistent with the time course expected of a process which awaits the development of delayed, non-reinforcing permeability changes (c.f. development of g_K during depolarizing clamps). The precipitous onset of the "off"-release suggests that the channels carrying the essential "releasing currents" are already open and transmitter release only awaits a change in membrane potential which will provide the driving force needed to move the "releasing currents" into the terminal.

These results will only become meaningful in the context of the "calcium hypothesis" if it can be shown that E_{RC} approximates to E_{Ca} i.e. the "releasing currents" are carried by Ca ions. Unfortunately, there is only limited data on the axoplasmic content of Ca ions and it is not possible to derive anything more than a very approximate value for E_{Ca}. Hodgkin & Keynes (1957) estimate that over 98 per cent of the calcium in the squid axon is bound in complex form and probably only 0·01 mmole/Kg.H_2O exists in a free, ionized state; with $[Ca]_o = 11$ mmole/Kg.H_2O, substitution in the Nernst Equation provides a value of about +90 mV for E_{Ca}. It remains to be seen if more accurate determinations of $[Ca]_i$ lead to a closer agreement between E_{Ca} and E_{RC}, but in the meantime it is difficult to see how any ion other than Ca could meet the requirements of the experimental data. It would be very interesting to know how E_{RC} is affected by changes in $[Ca]_o$ and clearly there will have to be further experiments before the "calcium hypothesis" is firmly accepted.

To summarise: the transmitter release is a delayed effect of depolarization, following in the wake of the invading nerve impulse. There is some evidence to suggest that the release is dependent upon a migration of Ca ions into the presynaptic terminal (the "releasing current"). This is probably achieved through changes in the permeability of the terminal membrane, and it is assumed that the transmitter release only proceeds when the Ca ions are established at critical "receptor" sites on the inner side of the membrane.

Functional Aspects of the Vertebrate Neuromuscular Junction

Functionally, the vertebrate nerve-muscle junction operates as a slave relay, the impulse traffic in the muscle being a "mirror image" of that in the motor nerve supplying it. Activation of the contractile elements is achieved by the uniform, self-reinforcing impulse which rapidly propagates throughout the muscle fibre and thereby synchronizes the shortening of its component parts. In the vertebrate locomotor system therefore, there is no peripheral modification of the central command signals and all movements are determined solely by the impulse traffic in the motor nerves.

Since there are far more muscle fibres than there are motoneurones, it is customary for groups of muscle fibres to share a common motor nerve. On reaching the muscle, each motor nerve terminal branches, often profusely, to innervate a number of muscle fibres, which as a result always act in concert. Thus, for the purpose of control, muscle fibres are organized into groups: each motoneurone plus the muscle fibres which it supplies compose *a motor unit*, which is the fundamental unit, or quantum, of muscle action. The tension developed in the muscle clearly depends upon the number of motor units involved, which in turn is a function of the activity in the motor nerve. In addition, the strength of contraction will be determined by the number of muscle fibres per motor unit—the innervation ratio—which can vary markedly from muscle to muscle. In the extrinsic eye muscles for instance, this ratio may be as low as 4 or 5, whilst in the large muscles of the leg it may be 150 or more. The magnitude of this ratio places a limit upon the delicacy with which muscles can be controlled. Thus, the low values characteristic of the eye muscles accord with their exacting control requirements whilst the high values found in the large postural muscles reflect more gross demands.

The Nervous Control of Crustacean Muscle

The nervous control of crustacean muscle is organized on a very different basis from the vertebrate system considered above. Each crustacean muscle fibre receives multiple excitatory and inhibitory inputs whose antagonistic effects on the membrane interact to determine the tension developed by the contractile elements. This integration of several converging inputs which occurs at the surface of the muscle fibre is very similar in many ways to the processing which takes place at the soma-dendritic membranes of neurones in the brain and spinal cord. The relative simplicity of the crustacean organization, together with its accessibility, have made it more amenable to investigation than the central neurones and a great deal has been learned from this system which has helped to elucidate some of the processing operations performed in the CNS.

A very striking feature of the crustacean nervous system is the immense paucity of motoneurones. This is particularly noticeable in the thoracic legs of the decapods where almost the whole musculature relies upon a mere handful of axons and two of the muscles—the opener and stretch muscles—actually share a single excitor axon (Hoyle & Wiersma, 1958a). Nonetheless, each muscle fibre enjoys a multiple innervation since the motor nerve divides and subdivides repeatedly, distributing axon terminals over the entire surface of each individual muscle fibre.

Impulses arriving in the excitatory terminals produce a local depolarization of the muscle membrane—*the excitatory junction potential* (e.j.p.)—which is very similar to the e.p.p. recorded at the vertebrate end-plates (Fatt & Katz, 1953b). However, most crustacean muscle fibres are relatively inexcitable in that they do not support self-regenerating impulses and rely entirely upon the local e.j.p.'s to activate the contractile elements. The multiple innervation enjoyed by each muscle fibre ensures that the depolarization is distributed throughout its entire length and thereby achieves synchrony in the shortening of the various elements. The spike activity supported by some crustacean muscle fibres loses much of its significance since the impulses arise simultaneously in all parts of the muscle, precluding the necessity for propagation. In these circumstances, the main role of the spike is to intensify and speed the onset of depolarization, hence accelerating the build-up of tension.

The tension developed in many crustacean muscle fibres is closely related to the membrane potential, and the strength of contraction is graded by manipulating this potential through modulation of the impulse traffic in the motor nerves (Hoyle & Wiersma, 1958c). Single shocks to the motor nerve produce very small e.j.p.'s and probably undetectable shortening. When repetitive pulses are applied, successive e.j.p.'s summate, each adding to the remnants of the previous one(s). The tension developed in the fibre reflects the mean level of depolarization achieved in this summation. Clearly, for effective summation, the interval between successive impulses should not exceed the duration of the e.j.p. With longer intervals (lower repetition rates), each e.j.p. decays before its successor commences and the result is simply a series of low-level e.j.p.'s. Thus, in general,

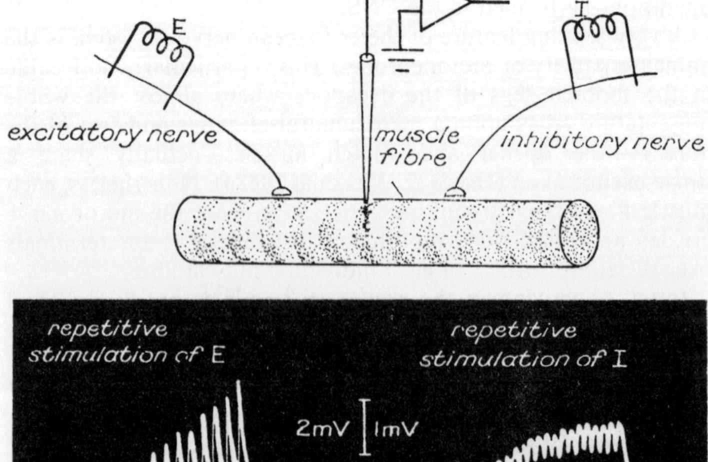

FIG. 74. Summation and facilitation of junction potentials at the crayfish muscle. When the excitatory and inhibitory nerves are stimulated repetitively (at 40 and 58 per second respectively), each junction potential adds on to the remnants of previous ones, thereby increasing the overall depolarization (summation). In addition, it is readily apparent that the individual junction potentials get progressively larger with each successive impulse due to augmented transmitter release probably caused by "residual" calcium in the presynaptic terminals (facilitation). Note that the i.j.p.'s are recorded at higher gain. (After Dudel & Kuffler, 1961b.)

the summation of e.j.p.'s becomes more complete as the inter-spike interval shortens, and the mean level of depolarization—and hence the strength of contraction—becomes a function of the impulse frequency in the motor nerve.

The transmitter substance at the crustacean nerve-muscle junction is known to be liberated in a quantal fashion (Dudel & Kuffler, 1961a) but the actual substance involved has not so far been identified although its effects can be mimiced with glutamate (Takeuki & Takeuki, 1964). The presumed permeability changes which give rise to the e.j.p. have not been investigated and it is not known exactly which ions are involved, though it seems safe to assume that Na ions play some part (Edwards, Terzuolo & Washizu, 1963).

Crustacean muscle also receives an inhibitory nerve supply, and fortunately, the excitatory and inhibitory axons to some muscles are contained in separate bundles, making it possible to study their effects on the postsynaptic membrane quite separately. Stimulation of the inhibitory nerve supply can cause relaxation of the muscle, regardless of any excitatory input (Fatt & Katz, 1953a; Hoyle & Wiersma, 1958b). Single inhibitory impulses produce small changes in the membrane potential of the muscle fibre—*the inhibitory junction potentials* (i.j.p.'s)—and though stimulation in high frequency bursts causes summation of these i.j.p.'s the total change in membrane potential is limited to a few millivolts.

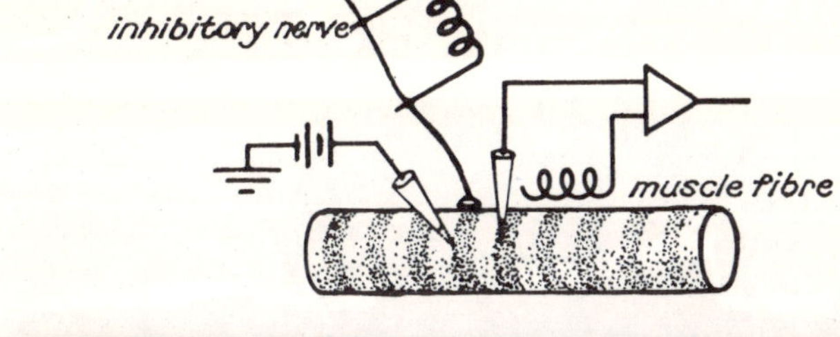

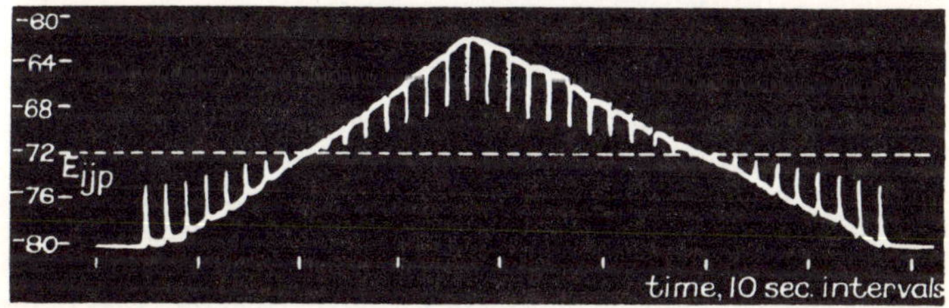

Fig. 75. The equilibrium potential for the inhibitory currents at the crayfish neuromuscular junction. Short trains of stimuli to the inhibitory nerve (at 150 per second) were repeated every 2 seconds whilst E_m was steadily displaced to new levels by passing current from a second intracellular electrode. The i.j.p.'s consistently shift E_m toward − 72mV, the equilibrium potential for the inhibitory currents: E_{ijp}. (After Dudel & Kuffler, 1961c.)

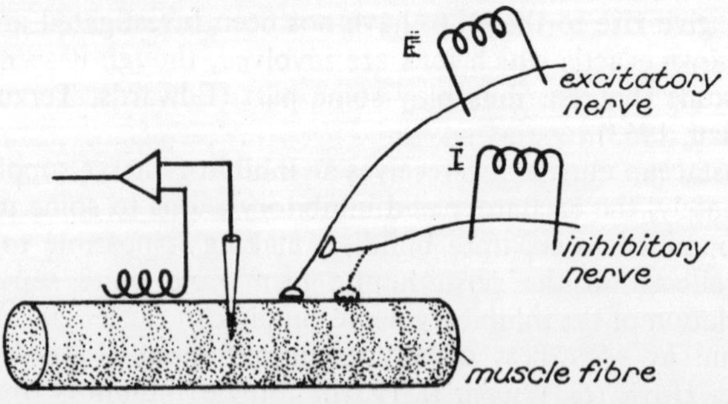

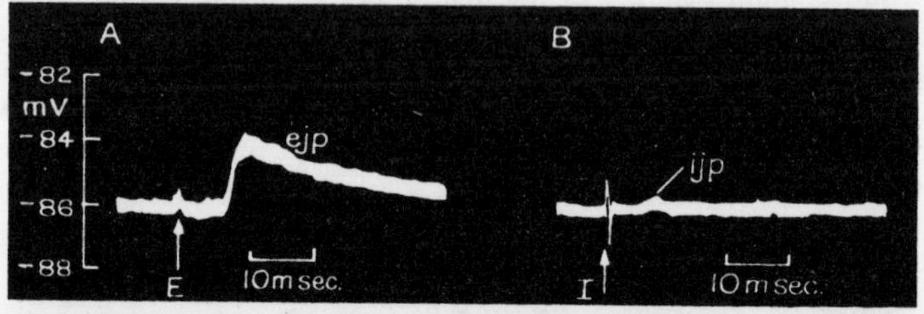

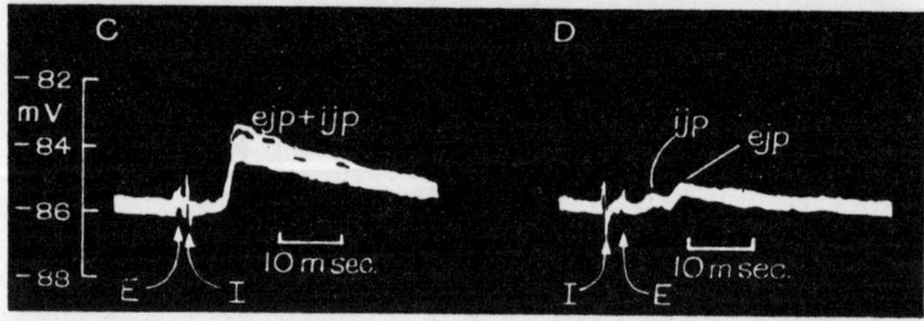

FIG. 76. Presynaptic inhibition at the crayfish neuromuscular junction. A: a single e.j.p. following stimulation of the excitatory nerve at *E*. B: a single i.j.p. following stimulation of the inhibitory nerve at I, with transmitter release on to the postsynaptic surface from the terminal in dotted line. C: an excitatory stimulus is followed by an inhibitory stimulus with an interval of 1·5 msec so that the peaks of the e.j.p. and i.j.p. coincide and actually summate in this particular instance. (Note that in this preparation, E_{ijp} (− 80mV) was on the depolarizing side of the resting potential which had been artificially raised to − 86mV by reducing $[K]_o$, hence summation of e.j.p. and i.j.p.) D: the inhibitory axon was stimulated 3 msec before the excitatory axon, giving rise to a normal i.j.p. which precedes a greatly reduced e.j.p. This potent suppression of the e.j.p. is due to inhibitory

Intracellular recordings from the muscle show that these i.j.p.'s result from a transient rise in membrane conductance. Dudel & Kuffler (1961c) recorded i.j.p.'s from the crayfish neuromuscular junction and investigated the effect of displacing membrane potential with current from a second microelectrode (see Fig. 75). These studies revealed that activation of the inhibitory input always shifts membrane potential towards −72 mV and the i.j.p. shows a sharp reversal in "polarity" at this potential. Thus, −72 mV represents the reversal potential for the inhibitory currents (E_{ijp}), strongly suggesting that the channels opened up by the inhibitory transmitter carry ion(s) which are close to equilibrium in the resting muscle i.e. K and/or Cl ions. The experiments of Boistel & Fatt (1958) indicate that the Cl-channels carry most of the inhibitory currents. Clearly, the inhibitory input protects the resting potential against any considerable changes by short-circuiting the membrane with low-resistance Cl-channels. E_{Cl} must approximate to E_{ijp} (i.e. −72 mV) and deviations in membrane potential away from this level will generate restoring forces on the Cl ions. Accordingly, the depolarizing effects of the excitatory input will be opposed by Cl-fluxes through the "inhibitory channels" whenever the inhibitory nerves are active.

Boistel & Fatt were able to mimic all of the inhibitory effects by administering the drug, gamma-aminobutyric acid (GABA) and there is now substantial evidence suggesting that this substance is the inhibitory transmitter at several crustacean synapses (Otsuka, Iverson, Hall & Kravitz, 1966).

The inhibition described above is often called *postsynaptic inhibition* because it operates by modifying the *post*synaptic membrane. Dudel & Kuffler (1961c) have demonstrated another inhibitory process at the crustacean nerve-muscle junction which modifies the membranes of the *pre*synaptic, excitatory terminals and hence is termed *presynaptic inhibition*. These workers found that often the i.j.p.'s following stimulation of the inhibitory nerve could actually precede the arrival of an excitatory input to the muscle and yet there would still be a marked reduction in the subsequent e.j.p. (see Fig. 76). Such "inhibition" cannot be explained by the process discussed above since it persists after the normal

endings on the excitatory terminals: presynaptic inhibition. Note that all records show several superimposed traces to provide an average response. (After Dudel & Kuffler, 1961c.)

postsynaptic process is concluded. However, this experiment tells us little about the nature of the "new" process. In this respect, Dudel & Kuffler made the very revealing discovery that the e.j.p. was reduced because the excitatory terminals liberated fewer quanta of the transmitter substance i.e. the inhibition is due to an effect on the *pre*synaptic, excitatory terminals and hence the term *pre*synaptic inhibition.

It will be realized that the two inhibitory mechanisms achieve very similar ends by two quite different means: both reduce the efficacy of the excitatory input to the muscle, the one by reducing the presynaptic release of the excitatory transmitter substance and the other by reducing its postsynaptic effect on the membrane potential of the muscle fibre. The necessity for two different inhibitory mechanisms is obscure, but the fact that they appear "in parallel" gives some basis for supposing that their effects are complementary.

It is not known exactly how the presynaptic inhibitory endings reduce the output of transmitter substance from excitatory terminals, and technically the problem presents considerable difficulties since the fine presynaptic terminals are too narrow for intracellular recording. Possibly the simplest of the explanations which can be offered to account for presynaptic inhibition assumes that the characteristic suppression of excitatory transmitter release is accomplished through a reduction in the amplitude of the excitatory spike. It has already been seen that transmitter release is very sensitive to changes in the size of the terminal spike (p. 104). Thus, any mechanism which modifies the terminal membrane in a way which will short-circuit or reduce the action currents, will compromise both the spike and the transmitter release which depends upon it. Of course, the short-circuit could be simply a non-specific rise in membrane conductance, or alternatively, merely a rise in P_K and/or P_{Cl} (Dudel, 1965a). (It is interesting in this respect that GABA—which mimics *post*synaptic inhibition and opens up Cl-channels in the muscle membrane—can also mimic the effects of *pre*synaptic inhibition (Dudel, 1965b). However, much more rigorous investigations are necessary before GABA can be accepted as the substance which normally mediates *pre*synaptic inhibition. Even so, there is no guarantee that GABA operates on the same ionic channels at the two different sites.) A non-specific rise in membrane conductance would most probably lead to some depolarization of the terminals which would have the added effect of raising the level of g_{Na}-inactivation and hence reducing the channels available for the action currents.

The tension in each crustacean muscle fibre accords with the balance of activity in its excitatory and inhibitory nerves. Thus, the crustacean neuromuscular system possesses an integrative ability which is in sharp contrast with the slave relay function of its vertebrate counterpart. The vertebrate of course, performs all of its processing operations within the CNS.

Central Synapses

The advent of intracellular recording techniques using micropipettes has led to considerable advances in our knowledge of central synapses and the mechanisms governing their function. Major contributors in this field have been Eccles and his co-workers, who recorded from the cell bodies of motoneurones in the spinal cord of the cat. Probably more is known about the synaptic processes at the surface of these spinal motoneurones than at any other site in the vertebrate CNS and this summary account will be restricted in the main to these synapses. Many of the basic mechanisms closely resemble those already encountered in crustacean muscle.

The Excitatory Postsynaptic Potential (e.p.s.p.). When a microelectrode penetrates the cell body of a spinal motoneurone, the oscilloscope indicates an immediate drop in potential of about 70 mV in a good preparation. Since the cell body may be subject to the tonic influence of excitatory and/or inhibitory impulses, it is difficult to be certain that this represents a true "resting" potential, but for the sake of simplicity, we will assume it to be so. The cell can be identified as a motoneurone supplying a particular muscle by the appearance of an antidromic spike on stimulation of the appropriate muscle nerve. Stimulation of the afferent fibres coming from that same muscle results in the synaptic excitation of the motoneurone and may lead to the generation of a spike (see Fig. 77).

The rising phase of the postsynaptic impulse often shows two inflexions, the lower one resulting from a synaptic potential which, like the e.p.p., is generated by transmitter action at the input terminals to the cell. If the strength of the stimulus is reduced then fewer afferent fibres are activated, the main spike fails to develop and only the so-called *excitatory postsynaptic potential* (e.p.s.p.) is recorded. This e.p.s.p. results from local

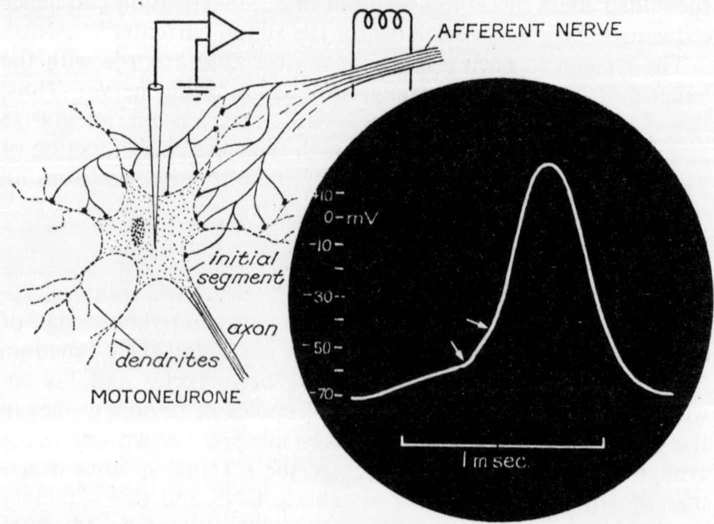

FIG. 77. An intracellular recording from a cat motoneurone during stimulation of an excitatory input. Note the inflexions in the rising phase of the spike potential: the first part is the subthreshold synaptic potential, the e.p.s.p., which traverses the cell body electrotonically and initiates an impulse in the membrane of the initial segment (first arrow); as this IS-spike develops, it depolarizes the soma beyond threshold (second arrow) and initiates an impulse there which "back-fires" into the dendrites. Meanwhile, the impulse also invades the axon and spreads to the periphery. (After Coombs, Curtis & Eccles, 1957a.)

transmitter action at the membrane beneath the excitatory terminals and is a non-regenerative response which attenuates rapidly with distance. It represents the normal synaptic mechanism by which incoming signals generate activity in the post-synaptic neurone (c.f. the e.p.p.).

The recorded e.p.s.p. is a composite potential which arises from activity in several presynaptic terminals, each of which creates a local depolarization. The tip of the recording electrode can be assumed to reside within the cell body—the dendrites being too narrow to penetrate—so that it will pick up the summated effects of terminals scattered over the cell body and its dendrites. The presynaptic endings are very small in comparison with the soma-

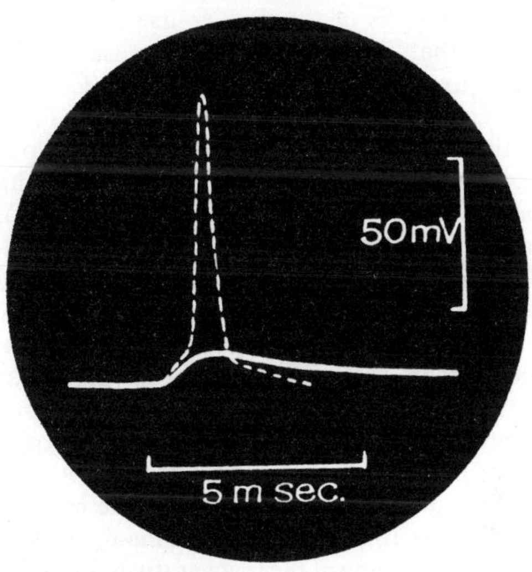

FIG. 78. The excitatory postsynaptic potential (e.p.s.p.) recorded intracellulary from a cat mononeurone in response to weak stimulation of an excitatory input. When only a few excitatory fibres are activated, the response is limited to a local e.p.s.p. which fails to depolarize the initial segment to threshold and hence fails to initiate any spike activity. The discontinuous line indicates the time course of the spike which develops when stronger stimuli are applied. (After Coombs, Curtis & Eccles, 1957b.)

dendritic membrane on which they impinge and the transmitter released from the individual terminals probably only modifies a minute proportion of this postsynaptic membrane. Thus, in order to drive the postsynaptic neurone beyond threshold and trigger a spike, there must be synchronous activity at a number of its inputs.

It seems likely that the presynaptic fibres which terminate out on the dendrites will tend to contribute less towards the recorded e.p.s.p. than similar endings near at hand on the cell body. Indeed, the depolarization produced in some of these dendrites may attenuate so severely that the recording system fails to detect them at all. Clearly, the irregular geometry of the soma-dendritic membrane must have a considerable influence upon the form of any intracellular recordings. We shall touch upon the functional significance of this spatial organization shortly.

An extensive analysis of the time course of many intracellular spikes suggests that the postsynaptic impulse originates in the first part of the axon, called *the initial segment* (Coombs, Curtis & Eccles, 1957a&b; Terzuolo & Araki, 1961; Araki & Terzuolo, 1962). This means that in order to evoke an impulse, the e.p.s.p. must be large enough to set up an electrotonic potential which extends beyond the cell body into the initial segment. Thus, the first inflexion in the rising phase of the postsynaptic impulse probably indicates the threshold in the initial segment, the soma-dendritic membrane being effectively "bypassed" because of a high threshold. However, the developing spike then propagates in both directions away from the initial segment i.e. as well as travelling out towards the muscle, the spike depolarizes the soma-dendritic membrane beyond its high threshold and hence "backfires" into the cell (c.f. impulse generation in the crayfish stretch receptor). The second inflexion in the rising phase of the intracellular spike probably marks the threshold in the soma-dendritic membrane and indicates the beginning of the regenerative spike in the cell body.

If these ideas on impulse genesis are correct then the cell body can be regarded as a relatively inexcitable receiving area, capable of handling large numbers of input signals at any given time. The initial segment functions as a remote sensor of this input traffic and is therefore unlikely to be triggered accidently by minor disturbances. An important factor which stems from this arrangement is that the geometrical location of the individual presynaptic endings—in particular, their proximity to the initial segment—will determine to a large extent the magnitude of their contributions to the activity of the postsynaptic neurone. This could well mean that some inputs are more influential than others and signals arriving at such endings would in effect enjoy priority over less well-situated inputs.

FIG. 79. The equilibrium potential for the e.p.s.p. at a cat motoneurone. A double-micropipette technique was employed to allow the recordings of e.p.s.p.'s with one barrel to proceed whilst currents were passed down the other to displace membrane potential to new levels. The e.p.s.p. always tends to shift membrane potential towards 0mV (E_{epsp}). Note that the individual membrane potentials are indicated by the position of the trace on the vertical scale and each record is formed by 20 superimposed responses. Time markers: 0·1 msec. (After Coombs, Eccles & Fatt, 1955b.)

afferent nerve
motoneurone
mV
+40
+30
+20
+10
0
Eepsp
-10
-20
-30
-40
-50
-60
resting potential
-70
-80

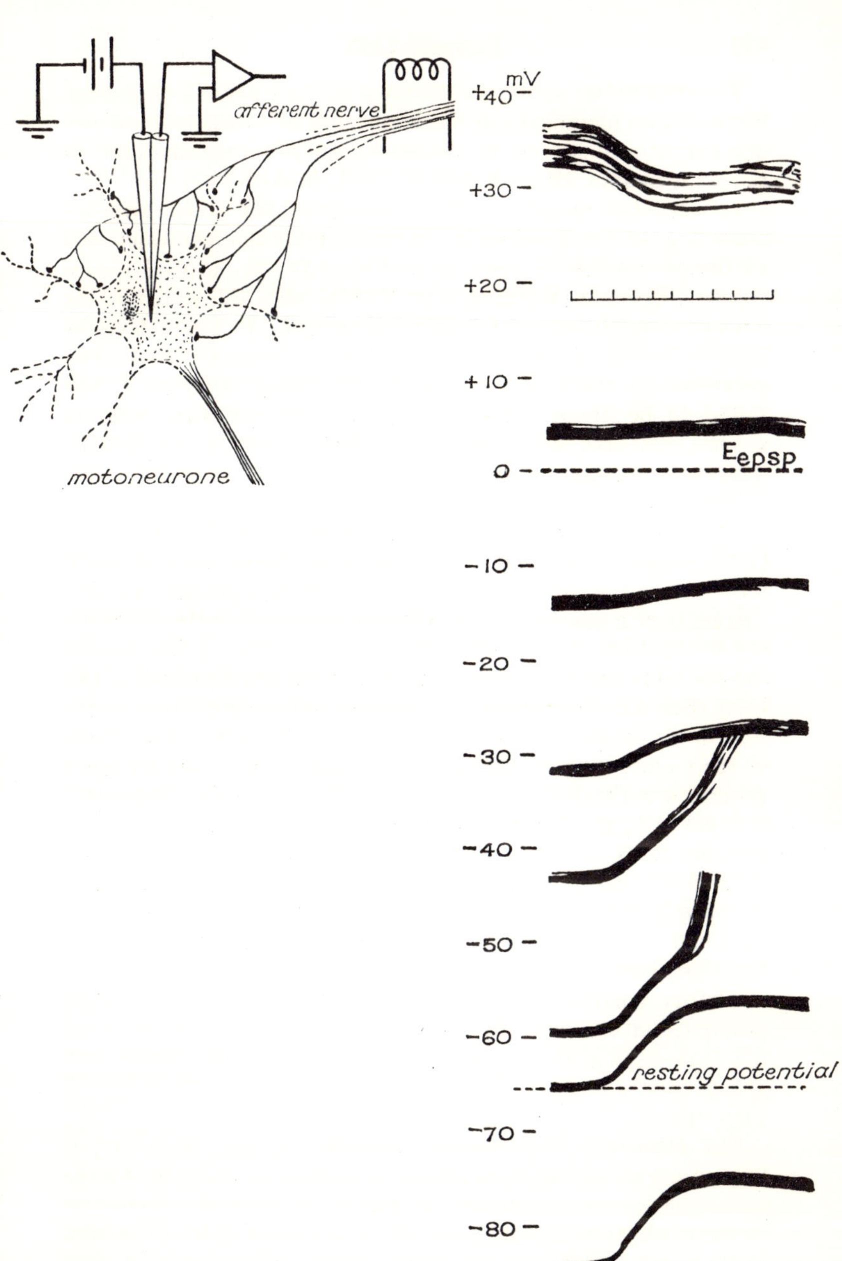

E.C.

The transmitter substance liberated at these excitatory endings has not been identified but the occurrence of small, spontaneous depolarizations similar to miniature e.p.p.'s suggests that its release is quantal (Katz & Miledi, 1963; Burke, 1967).

Intracellular recordings have also provided some evidence regarding the ions involved in the permeability changes which lead to the production of the e.p.s.p. Using double-barreled micropipettes, Coombs, Eccles & Fatt (1955b) were able to record the e.p.s.p. through one barrel after adjusting E_m to a new level by passing current through the other. By this means, the reversal potential for the ionic mechanism generating the e.p.s.p. was found to be about 0 mV. This, and other evidence, seem to suggest that the excitatory transmitter causes a non-specific increase in membrane permeability.

The reversal potential for the currents generating the e.p.s.p. is often difficult to demonstrate and Smith, Wuerker & Frank (1967) suggest that this could be due to excitatory endings which terminate out on the dendrites. These workers argue that passing current from a microelectrode whose tip is located in the cell body, is unlikely to be equally effective in adjusting the E_m throughout the cell body and the remote branches of the dendritic tree. If this is so, then the electrochemical gradients and driving forces on the ions in the dendrites will remain almost unaltered by adjustments in the membrane potential at the cell body. Thus, any e.p.s.p.'s generated in the dendrites will be little affected by the "apparent" changes in E_m produced by passing current from a microelectrode and, in particular, will probably not "reverse". Smith *et al.*, showed that, in their hands at least, the double-barrel technique could only detect conductance changes during the e.p.s.p. in less than half of their preparations. They attributed the failures to the fact that their electrode tips were situated too far away from the excitatory synapses i.e. the latter were dendritic. This supposed failure to detect remote inputs at the cell body raises the functional question of signal priorities once again—certain inputs will always exert a more profound influence on the activity of the cell than others.

The Inhibitory Postsynaptic Potential (i.p.s.p.). Some input fibres exert an inhibitory influence on the motoneurone, tending to reduce its firing rate. Intracellular recordings show that activation of these inhibitory inputs promotes a transient hyperpolarization of the soma, driving the cell away from its firing threshold. This

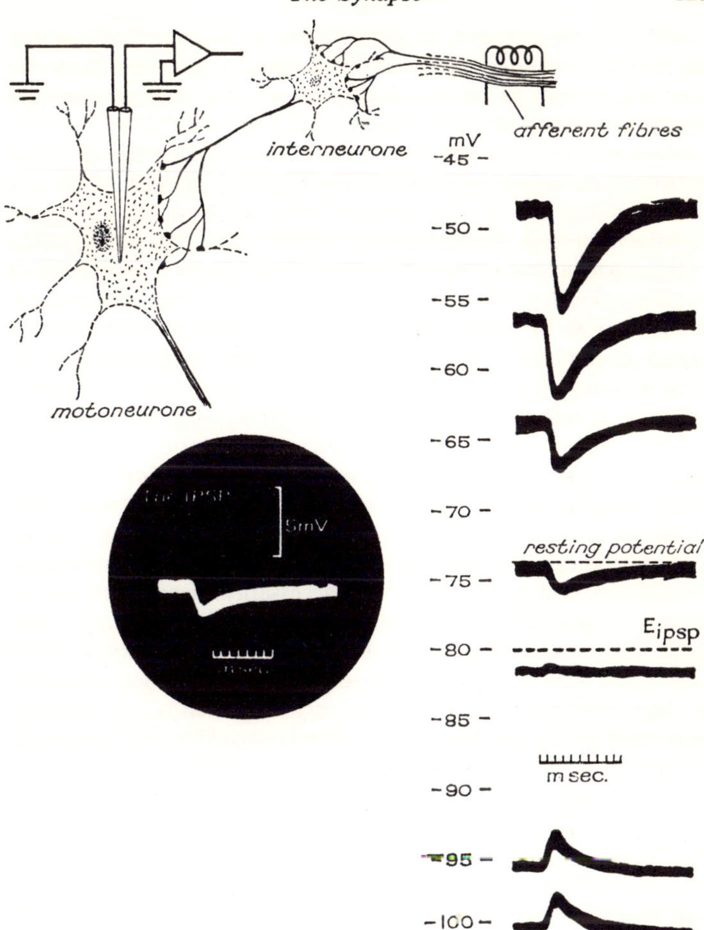

FIG. 80. The equilibrium potential for the i.p.s.p. at a cat motoneurone. The inset tracing shows the time course of the i.p.s.p. following a single stimulus to a suitable input. The multiple traces were made using one side of a double-micropipette whilst displacing membrane potential with current passed down the other. Again, the membrane potential in each instance is given by the position of the tracing on the vertical scale. Note that activation of the inhibitory input tends to drive the membrane potential towards $-$ 80mV (E_{ipsp}) and hence opposes any movement towards the firing threshold. (After Coombs, Eccles & Fatt, 1955a.)

local, synaptic potential is graded, rarely exceeds 5 mV and is called the *inhibitory postsynaptic potential* (i.p.s.p.). Using the double-micropipette technique to record i.p.s.p.'s at different membrane potentials, Coombs, Eccles & Fatt (1955a) found the reversal potential for the inhibitory currents to be some 10 mV greater than the resting potential, i.e. $E_{ipsp} = -80$ mV.

The finding that E_{ipsp} is close to the resting potential suggests that the inhibitory transmitter operates by raising the conductance of the postsynaptic membrane to ions which are near equilibrium in the resting nerve i.e. K ions and/or Cl ions. Eccles, Eccles & Ito (1964a & b) applied ion injection techniques to cat motoneurones and concluded that the inhibitory currents are carried by both K ions and Cl ions.

The reversal potential for the inhibitory currents is readily demonstrable and not subject to the uncertainties encountered with the excitatory currents. Smith *et al.*, (1967) found that in their experiments the i.p.s.p. was always associated with conductance changes and, applying the earlier arguments, this would seem to indicate that most of the inhibitory endings were located on the cell body. (This does not necessarily mean there are no inhibitory endings—from other sources—on the dendrites.) Once again this raises the question of the spatial distribution of the various synapses on the soma-dendritic membrane. Inhibitory endings which border the initial segment, such as those under investigation in the above experiments, would seem well poised to prevent any e.p.s.p.'s gaining entry to this vital part of the cell. However, although such endings could exert a very potent effect, it would be rather gross and indiscriminate, blocking a multitude of excitatory inputs without consideration for their source. Clearly, such coarse control of the processing operations in the cell is best reserved for only the most serious contingencies, the routine data handling being carried out more peripherally, i.e. on the dendrites. Such considerations however, at the present time rest largely on postulates and plausible suggestions.

Presynaptic Inhibition. Frank & Fuortes (1957) and Frank (1959) reported a form of inhibition in which the e.p.s.p. was suppressed in the absence of any detectable i.p.s.p. The failure to record an i.p.s.p. is not necessarily incompatible with a postsynaptic mechanism since this could happen if for one reason or another, $E_m = E_{ipsp}$. However, according to Eccles (1964) shifting E_m still fails to reveal any i.p.s.p. The inhibition must

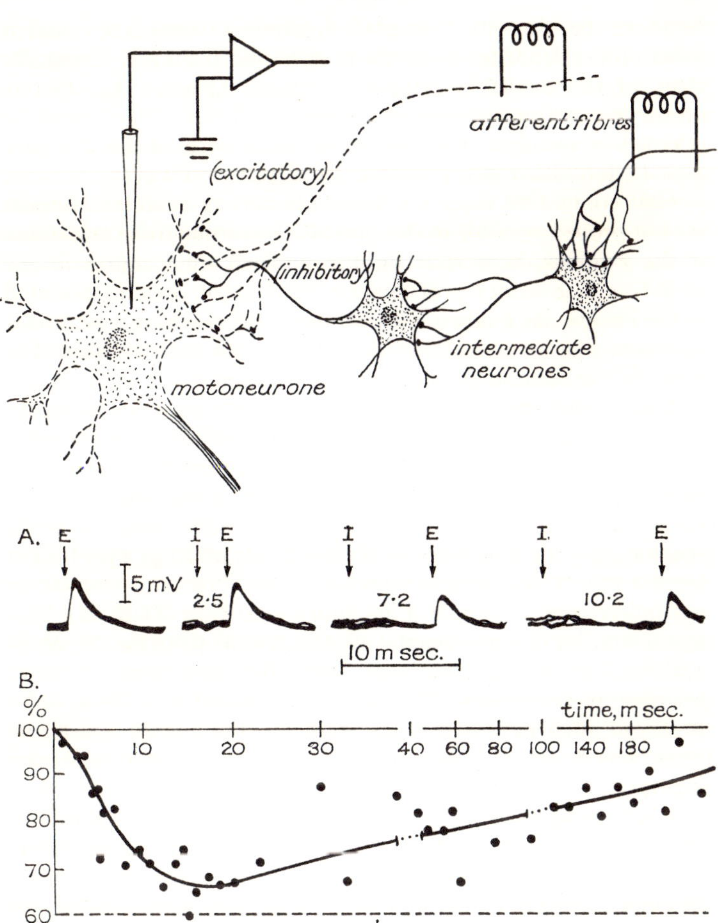

FIG. 81. Prolonged depression of monosynaptic e.p.s.p.'s. A: intracellular recordings from a motoneurone. The first tracing (control) shows the e.p.s.p. generated by a standard volley in an appropriate afferent nerve. Subsequent traces show the partial suppression of this e.p.s.p. by prior stimulation of other afferents at time intervals indicated by the figures over each tracing (in msec). B: the time course of the e.p.s.p. depression. Ordinate: e.p.s.p.'s as a percentage of the control. Abscissae: interval between conditioning and test volleys. Note that the suppression is maximal after some 15–20 msec and persists for over 200 msec. (Eccles, Eccles & Magni, 1961.)

therefore be due to "remote" inhibitory terminals, located either on the dendrites or on the presynaptic excitatory terminals. Most of the available evidence strongly suggests that this is another case of presynaptic inhibition.

You will recollect that the crucial piece of evidence for presynaptic inhibition in the crustacean preparation was the reduced quantal content of the e.j.p. Unfortunately, a similar approach has not proved possible in the case of the motoneurone and much of the evidence here rests on the unusual time course of the inhibition. The normal postsynaptic inhibitory process represented by the i.p.s.p. has a relatively brief duration, reaching a peak in a millisecond or so and usually decaying in less than 10 msec. The "remote" inhibition is much more prolonged (at least in cat motoneurones) taking about 20 msec. merely to reach its peak, and having an overall duration in excess of 200 msec (Eccles, Eccles & Magni, 1961). Intracellular recordings from incoming (presynaptic) fibres traversing the dorsum of the spinal cord—where the axon diameters are sufficient for microelectrode penetration—reveal that some of these fibres undergo a prolonged depolarization which coincides with the "remote" inhibition and indeed runs a parallel time course (see Figs. 81 & 82). This demonstration of a presynaptic event accompanying the "remote" inhibition invites comparisons with the presynaptic process described in crustaceans. On this basis, it would be quite in order to record such depolarizations from the presynaptic excitatory fibres which are assumed to be the target for the inhibitory endings.

Other experiments have shown that this "remote" inhibition is also associated with a drop in the threshold of the excitatory terminals (Eccles, Magni & Willis, 1962). It seems unlikely that the close correspondence between the time relations of these three events—depression of e.p.s.p.'s, depolarization of the afferent fibres and lowered threshold of the afferent terminals—could be fortuitous, and taken together they argue strongly in favour of presynaptic mechanisms. Similar observations have now been made at several different sites in the vertebrate nervous system.

From the functional point of view, presynaptic inhibition constitutes a potentially more specific and local phenomenon than the postsynaptic process. It provides a mechanism by which individual inputs can be "taken out of the reckoning" whilst others go forward for processing unimpeded. It is surely signifi-

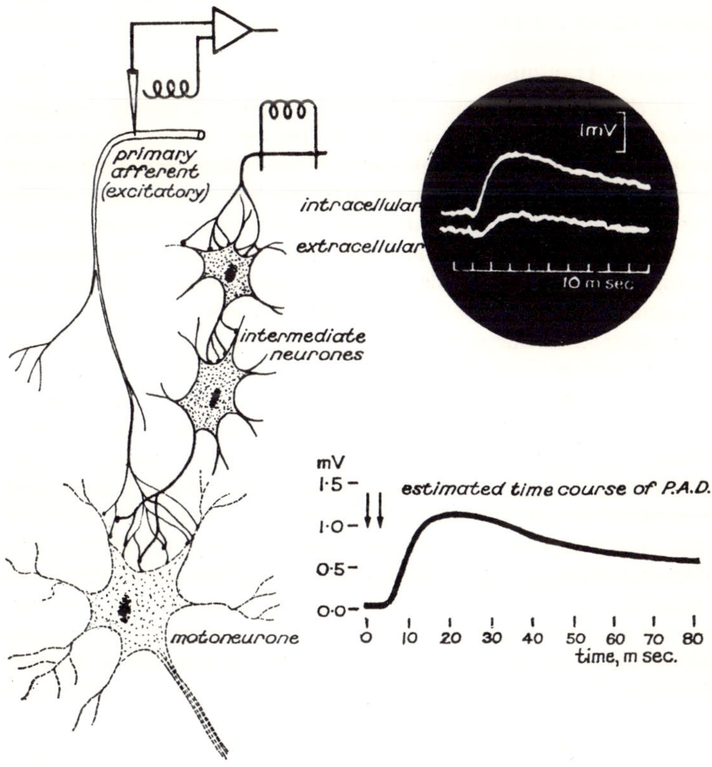

FIG. 82. The primary afferent depolarization (PAD). The inset shows the PAD resulting from two afferent volleys, recorded intracellularly (upper trace) and when the microelectrode is just withdrawn to an extracellular position (lower trace). The time course of the potential changes across the afferent nerve membrane is represented by the difference between these two recordings and is shown in the graph. (The arrows indicate the application of stimuli.) Note that the PAD is maximal after some 20 msec or so and persists for well over 80 msec. Such a time course closely parallels that of the e.p.s.p. depression seen in the previous figure, suggesting that both are part of the same phenomenon: presynaptic inhibition. (After Eccles, Magni & Willis, 1962.)

cant that presynaptic inhibition features in most of the cat's sensory systems, where it is well placed to assist in the selection of input signals for processing.*

Electrical Transmission

Work on invertebrate material has revealed several synapses where effective transfer occurs in the absence of a chemical transmitter. Such junctions seem to offer little resistance to the local circuit currents responsible for the normal transmission in the axon and adequate charge crosses the cleft to trigger activity in the postsynaptic neurone. Although many of these *electrical synapses* are very simple and permit transmission in either direction, others possess a rectifying property which restricts transmission to one direction only. A good example of a "rectifying" synapse is found in the crayfish nerve cord where giant lateral fibres synapse with the large segmental motor axons which pass out to the "tail" muscle. Furshpan & Potter (1959) made intracellular recordings on both sides of this synapse simultaneously and investigated the transmission of impulses which were generated by passing currents through additional, intracellular microelectrodes (see Fig. 83). Stimulation of the lateral fibre led to the appearance of an impulse in the motor fibre after a very brief delay of only 0·1 msec. On the other hand, stimulation of the motor fibre produced only a minute depolarization in the lateral giant fibre. Clearly, this is unidirectional transmission, with impulses passing only from the lateral giant (pre-) fibre to the motor (post-) fibre. Electron microscopy shows that the synaptic cleft at electrical synapses is much narrower than at chemical synapses, with the pre- and postsynaptic membrane actually fusing in certain areas (Robertson, 1955, 1961; de Lorenzo, 1959; Hama, 1961). However, the structural basis of the rectifying action has not been established.

Most nerve fibres are filled with, and surrounded by, a good conducting medium. The currents associated with nervous activity therefore, flow freely through the axoplasm and external medium and almost the whole of the voltage gradient associated with the

---

*Mendell & Wall (1964) have demonstrated that some inputs to the spinal cord can *hyperpolarize* certain presynaptic terminals and hence amplify the impulses arriving in such endings. This process has been termed *presynaptic facilitation* and clearly has effects which are diametrically opposite to those of the inhibitory presynaptic process described above.

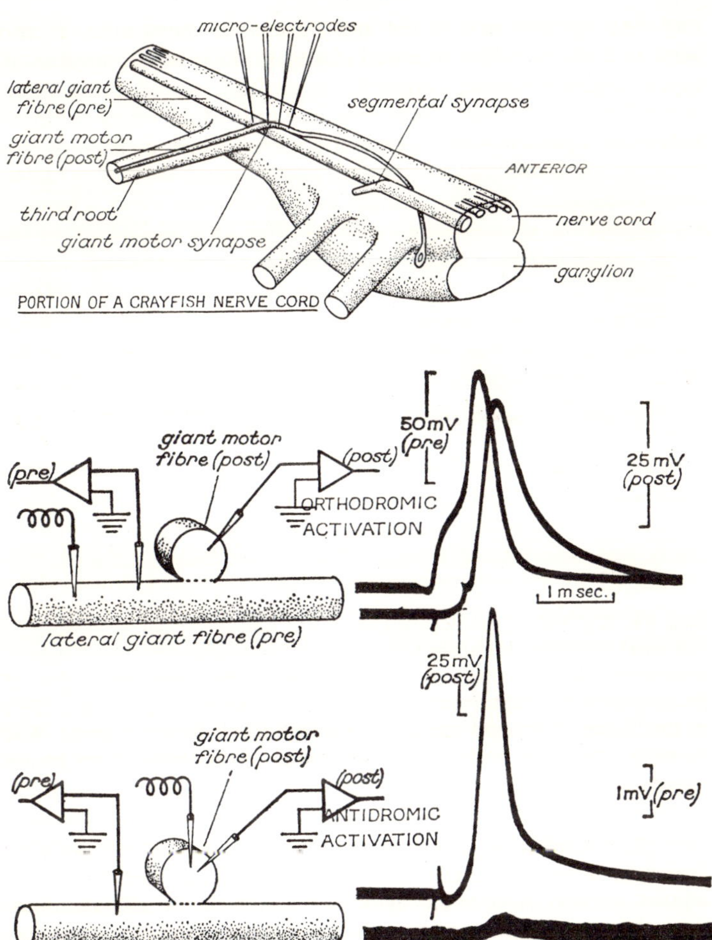

FIG. 83. The rectifying electrical synapse in the crayfish abdominal nerve cord. Upper trace: shows orthodromic transmission from the lateral giant fibre to the giant motor fibre with an almost negligible delay. Lower trace: failure of antidromic transmission; the response in the lateral giant fibre is very low level even though the recording gain is very high. Note that directly stimulated structures (and their responses) are shown in red whilst trans-synaptically activated ones are in green. (After Furshpan & Potter, 1959.)

impulses appears across the high-resistance membrane. If this were not so, then the potential changes which would appear in, say, a high-resistance, extracellular medium would cause interaction between adjacent neurones, and individual axons could no longer be regarded as independent channels. Such a situation has

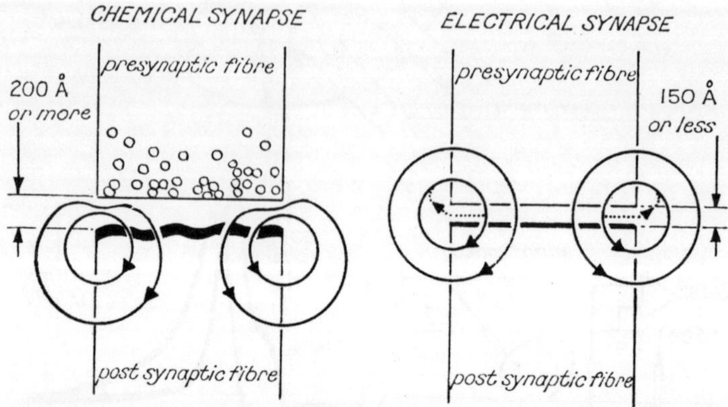

FIG. 84. A comparison between chemical and electrical synapses. At chemical synapses, impulses are set up in the postsynaptic structure as a result of depolarizing currents consequent to transmitter action at the postsynaptic membrane. At electrical synapses, the synaptic cleft is much narrower and permits sufficient local circuit current flow between pre- and postsynaptic structures to maintain propagation across the junction.

FIG. 85. Electrical inhibition at the Mauthner cell of the goldfish. Traces A, B and D are intracellular recordings and trace C is extracellular; all were made in the region of the axon cap. A: stimulation of the eighth cranial nerve (at E) generates a spike in the Mauthner cell. B: stimulation at E is preceded by antidromic activation of the contralateral Mauthner cell axon at I. The latter activates a collateral pathway which raises the threshold for spike initiation (as indicated by the arrows) and hence inhibits the Mauthner cell. C: shows the extrinsic hyperpolarizing potential (EHP) resulting from activation of the collateral inhibitory pathway alone. It is this potential which elevates the spike threshold. D: is an intracellular recording which reveals late chemical inhibition (in the form of an i.p.s.p.) following activation of the collateral pathway and transmitter release at the inhibitory terminals. (After Furukawa & Furshpan, 1963.)

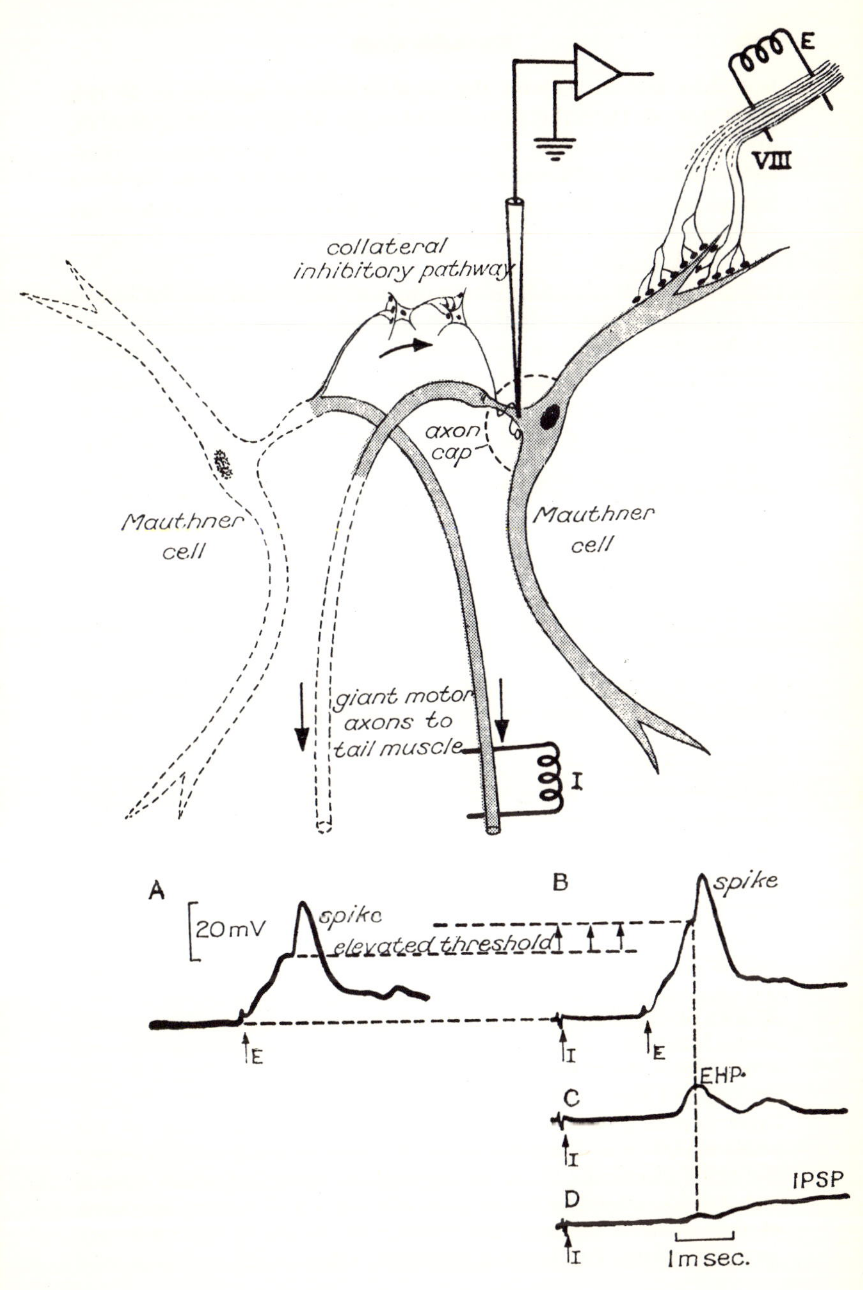

E
VIII
collateral
inhibitory pathway
axon
cap
Mauthner
cell
Mauthner
cell
giant motor
axons to
tail muscle
I
A
20 mV
spike
elevated threshold
E
B
spike
I
E
C
EHP
I
D
IPSP
I
1 m sec.

been found to exist in the region of the initial segment of certain giant cells in the fish brain. These large, Mauthner cells, as they are called, receive numerous chemical synaptic endings on their soma-dendritic membrane but our only concern is with the axon hillock, which is invested with densely packed glia and thin axons which terminate in helical coils. The whole mass forms the *axon cap* (see Fig. 85).

Extracellular recordings from the axon cap reveal that the action currents associated with impulses arriving in these helical terminals produce large, positive potentials (10 to 15 mV), presumably as a result of the high resistance of this region. Intracellular recordings from the Mauthner cell show that the initial segment is hyperpolarized by these currents, thus raising the threshold for impulse initiation in the neurone. This *electrical inhibition* has not been demonstrated elsewhere as yet, but there are several sites familiar to the histologist which show similar structural arrangements. It remains to be seen if effective inhibition occurs in these other regions or whether the Mauthner cell is unique.

BIBLIOGRAPHY

ADRIAN, R. H. (1960). Potassium chloride movement and the membrane potential of frog muscle. *J. Physiol.* **151,** 154.

ADRIAN, R. H. (1961). Internal chloride concentration and chloride efflux of frog muscle. *J. Physiol.* **156,** 623.

ARAKI, T. & TERZUOLO, C. A. (1962). Membrane currents in spinal motoneurons associated with the action potential and synaptic activity. *J. Neurophysiol.* **25,** 772.

BAKER, P. F., HODGKIN, A. L. & SHAW, T. I. (1962). Replacement of the axoplasm of giant nerve fibres with artificial solutions. *J. Physiol.* **164,** 330.

BIRKS, R., HUXLEY, H. E. & KATZ, B. (1960). The fine structure of the neuromuscular junction of the frog. *J. Physiol.* **150,** 134.

BLOEDEL, J. R., GAGE, P. W., LLINAS, R. & QUASTEL, D. M. J. (1966). Transmitter release at the squid giant synapse in the presence of tetrodotoxin. *Nature, Lond.* **212,** 49.

BLOEDEL, J. R., GAGE, P. W., LLINAS, R. & QUASTEL, D.M.J. (1967). Transmission across the squid giant synapse in the presence of tetrodotoxin. *J. Physiol.* **188,** 52 P.

BODIAN, D. (1952). Introductory survey of neurons. *Cold Spring Harbor Symp. Quant. Biol.* **17,** 1.

BOISTEL, J. & FATT, P. (1958). Membrane permeability change during inhibitory transmitter action in crustacean muscle. *J. Physiol.* **144,** 176.

BOYD, I. A. & MARTIN, A. R. (1956). The end-plate potential in mammalian muscle. *J. Physiol.* **132,** 74.

BROCK, L. G., COOMBS, J. S. & ECCLES, J. C. (1952). The recording of potentials from motoneurones with an intracellular electrode. *J. Physiol.* **117,** 431.

BURKE, R. E. (1967). Composite nature of the monosynaptic excitatory postsynaptic potential. *J. Neurophysiol.* **30,** 1114.

CALDWELL, P. C., HODGKIN, A. L., KEYNES, R. D. & SHAW, T. I. (1960). The effects of injecting energy-rich phosphate compounds on the active transport of ions in the giant axons of *Loligo*. *J. Physiol.* **152,** 561.

COLE, K. S. (1949). Dynamic electrical characteristics of the squid axon membrane. *Arch. Sci. Physiol.* **3,** 253.

COLERIDGE, J. C. G. & KIDD, C. (1960). Electrophysiological evidence of baroreceptors in the pulmonary artery of the dog. *J. Physiol.* **150,** 319.

COOMBS, J. S., CURTIS, D. R. & ECCLES, J. C. (1957a). The interpretation of spike potentials of motoneurones. *J. Physiol.* **139,** 198.

COOMBS, J. S., CURTIS, D. R. & ECCLES, J. C. (1957b). The generation of impulses in motoneurones. *J. Physiol.* **139,** 232.

COOMBS, J. S., ECCLES, J. C. & FATT, P. (1955a). The specific ionic conductances and the ionic movements across the motoneuronal membrane that produce the inhibitory post-synaptic potential. *J. Physiol.* **130,** 326.

COOMBS, J. S., ECCLES, J. C. & FATT, P. (1955b). Excitatory synaptic action in motoneurones. *J. Physiol.* **130,** 374.

COWAN, S. L. (1940). The actions of eserine-like compounds upon frog's nerve-muscle preparations, and conditions in which a single shock can evoke an augmented muscular response. *Proc. R. Soc.* B **129,** 356.

CRAGG, B. G. (1967). The density of synapses and neurones in the motor and visual areas of the cerebral cortex. *J. Anat.* **101,** 639.

CROWE, A. & MATTHEWS, P. B. C. (1964). The effects of stimulation of static and dynamic fusimotor fibres on the response to stretching of the primary endings of muscle spindles. *J. Physiol.* **174,** 109.

DALE, H. H., FELDBERG, W. & VOGT, M. (1936). Release of acetylcholine at voluntary motor nerve endings. *J. Physiol.* **86,** 353.

DEL CASTILLO, J. & KATZ, B. (1954a). Quantal components of the end-plate potential. *J. Physiol.* **124,** 560.

DEL CASTILLO, J. & KATZ, B. (1954b). The membrane change produced by the neuromuscular transmitter. *J. Physiol.* **125,** 546.

DEL CASTILLO, J. & KATZ, B. (1955). On the localization of acetylcholine receptors. *J. Physiol.* **128,** 157.

DE LORENZO, A. J. (1959). The fine structure of synapses. *Biol. Bull.* **117,** 390.

DE ROBERTIS, E. (1964). Electron microscope and chemical study of binding sites of brain biogenic amines. *Progr. Brain Res.* **8,** 118.

DUDEL, J. (1965a). The mechanism of presynaptic inhibition at the crayfish neuromuscular junction. *Pflügers Arch. Ges. Physiol.* **284,** 66.

DUDEL, J. (1965b). The action of inhibitory drugs on nerve terminals in crayfish muscle. *Pflügers Arch. Ges. Physiol.* **284,** 81.

DUDEL, J. & KUFFLER, S. W. (1961a). The quantal nature of transmission and spontaneous miniature potentials at the crayfish neuromuscular junction. *J. Physiol.* **155,** 514.

DUDEL, J. & KUFFLER, S. W. (1961b). Mechanism of facilitation at the crayfish neuromuscular junction. *J. Physiol.* **155,** 530.

DUDEL, J. & KUFFLER, S. W. (1961c). Presynaptic inhibition at the crayfish neuromuscular junction. *J. Physiol.* **155,** 543.

ECCLES, J. C. (1964). *The Physiology of Synapses*, p. 221. Springer-Verlag OHG, Berlin.

ECCLES, J. C., ECCLES, R. M. & ITO, M. (1964a). Effects of intracellular potassium and sodium injections on the inhibitory postsynaptic potential. *Proc. R. Soc.* B **160,** 181.

ECCLES, J. C., ECCLES, R. M. & ITO, M. (1964b). Effects produced on inhibitory postsynaptic potentials by the coupled injections of cations and anions into motoneurones. *Proc. R. Soc.* B. **160,** 197.

ECCLES, J. C., ECCLES, R. M. & MAGNI, F. (1961). Central inhibitory action attributable to presynaptic depolarization produced by muscle afferent volleys. *J. Physiol.* **159,** 147.

ECCLES, J. C., MAGNI, F. & WILLIS, W. D. (1962). Depolarization of central terminals of Group I afferent fibres from muscle. *J. Physiol.* **160,** 62.

EDWARDS, C. & HAGIWARA, S. (1959). Potassium ions and the inhibitory process in the crayfish stretch receptor. *J. gen. Physiol.* **43,** 315.

EDWARDS, C. & OTTOSON, D. (1958). The site of impulse initiation in a nerve cell of a crustacean stretch receptor. *J. Physiol.* **143,** 138.

EDWARDS, C., TERZUOLO, C. A. & WASHIZU, Y. (1963). The effect of changes of the ionic environment upon an isolated crustacean sensory neuron. *J. Neurophysiol.* **26,** 948.

ELMQVIST, D. & FELDMAN, D. S. (1965). Spontaneous activity at a mammalian neuromuscular junction in tetrodotoxin. *Acta. physiol. scand.* **64,** 475.

EYZAGUIRRE, C. & KUFFLER, S. W. (1955). Processes of excitation in the dendrites and in the soma of single isolated sensory nerve cells of the lobster and crayfish. *J. gen. Physiol.* **39,** 87.

FATT, P. & KATZ, B. (1950). Some observations on biological noise. *Nature, Lond.* **166,** 597.

FATT, P. & KATZ, B. (1951). An analysis of the end-plate potential recorded with an intra-cellular electrode. *J. Physiol.* **115,** 320.

FATT, P. & KATZ, B. (1952). Spontaneous subthreshold activity at motor nerve endings. *J. Physiol.* **117,** 109.

FATT, P. & KATZ, B. (1953a). Distributed 'end-plate potentials' of crustacean muscle fibres. *J. exp. Biol.* **30,** 433.

FATT, P. & KATZ, B. (1953b). The effect of inhibitory nerve impulses on a crustacean muscle fibre. *J. Physiol.* **121,** 374.

FRANK, K. (1959). Basic mechanisms of synaptic transmission in the central nervous system. *I.R.E. Trans. Med. Electron.* **ME-6,** 85.

FRANK, K. & FUORTES, M. G. F. (1957). Presynaptic and postsynaptic inhibition of monosynaptic reflexes. *Fed. Proc.* **16,** 39.

FURSHPAN, E. J. & POTTER, D. D. (1959). Transmission at the giant motor synapses of the crayfish. *J. Physiol.* **145,** 289.

FURUKAWA, T. & FURSHPAN, E. J. (1963). Two inhibitory mechanisms in the Mauthner neurones of goldfish. *J. Neurophysiol.* **26,** 140.

FURUKAWA, T., SASAOKA, T. & HOSOYA, Y. (1959). Effects of tetrodotoxin on the neuromuscular junction. *Jap. J. Physiol.* **9,** 143.

HAGIWARA, S., KUSANO, K. & SAITO, S. (1960). Membrane changes in crayfish stretch receptor neuron during synaptic inhibition and under action of gamma-aminobutyric acid. *J. Neurophysiol.* **23,** 505.

HAMA, K. (1961). Some observations on the fine structure of the giant fibres of the crayfishes (*Cambarus virilis* and *Cambarus clarkii*) with special reference to the sub-microscopic organization of the synapses. *Anat. Rec.* **141,** 275.

HILLE, B. (1967). The selective inhibition of delayed potassium currents in nerve by tetraethylammonium ion. *J. gen. Physiol.* **50,** 1287.

HODGKIN, A. L. (1958). The Croonian Lecture: Ionic movements and electrical activity in giant nerve fibres. *Proc. R. Soc.* B **148,** 1.

HODGKIN, A. L. (1964). *The Conduction of the Nervous Impulse*, p. 74. Liverpool University Press, Liverpool.

HODGKIN, A. L. & HOROWICZ, P. (1959). Movements of Na and K in single muscle fibres. *J. Physiol.* **145,** 405.

HODGKIN, A. L. & HUXLEY, A. F. (1952a). Currents carried by sodium and potassium ions through the membrane of the giant axon of *Loligo*. *J. Physiol.* **116,** 449.

HODGKIN, A. L. & HUXLEY, A. F. (1952b). The components of membrane conductance in the giant axon of *Loligo*. *J. Physiol.* **116,** 473.

HODGKIN, A. L. & HUXLEY, A. F. (1952c). The dual effect of membrane potential on sodium conductance in the giant axon of *Loligo*. *J. Physiol.* **116,** 497.

HODGKIN, A. L. & HUXLEY, A. F. (1952d). A quantitative description of membrane current and its application to conduction and excitation in nerve. *J. Physiol.* **117,** 500.

HODGKIN, A. L., HUXLEY, A. F. & KATZ, B. (1952). Measurement of current-voltage relations in the membrane of the giant axon of *Loligo*. *J. Physiol.* **116,** 424.

HODGKIN, A. L. & KATZ, B. (1949). The effect of sodium ions on the electrical activity of the giant axon of the squid. *J. Physiol.* **108,** 37.

HODGKIN, A. L. & KEYNES, R. D. (1955a). Active transport of cations in giant axons from *Sepia* and *Loligo*. *J. Physiol.* **128,** 28.

HODGKIN, A. L. & KEYNES, R. D. (1955b). The potassium permeability of a giant nerve fibre. *J. Physiol.* **128,** 61.

HODGKIN, A. L. & KEYNES, R. D. (1957). Movements of labelled calcium in squid giant axons. *J. Physiol.* **138.** 253.

HOYLE, G. & WIERSMA, C. A. G. (1958a). Excitation at neuromuscular junctions in Crustacea. *J. Physiol.* **143,** 403.

Hoyle, G. & Wiersma, C. A. G. (1958b). Inhibition at neuromuscular junctions in Crustacea. *J. Physiol.* **143,** 426.

Hoyle, G. & Wiersma, C. A. G. (1958c). Coupling of membrane potential to contraction in crustacean muscles. *J. Physiol.* **143,** 441.

Hubbard, S. J. (1958). A study of rapid mechanical events in a mechanoreceptor. *J. Physiol.* **141,** 198.

Hutter, O. F. & Noble, D. (1960). The chloride conductance of frog skeletal muscle. *J. Physiol.* **151,** 89.

Karlsson, U. (1966). Three-dimensional studies of neurons in the lateral geniculate nucleus of the rat. II. Environment of perikarya and proximal parts of their branches. *J. Ultrastruc. Res.* **16,** 482.

Karlsson, U. (1967). Three-dimensional studies of neurons in the lateral geniculate nucleus of the rat. III. Specialized neuronal contacts in the neuropil. *J. Ultrastruc. Res.* **17,** 137.

Katz, B. & Miledi, R. (1963). A study of spontaneous miniature potentials in spinal motoneurones. *J. Physiol.* **168,** 389.

Katz, B. & Miledi, R. (1965a). Propagation of electric activity in motor nerve terminals. *Proc. R. Soc.* B **161,** 453.

Katz, B. & Miledi, R. (1965b). The measurement of synaptic delay, and the time course of acetylcholine release at the neuromuscular junction. *Proc. R. Soc.* B **161,** 483.

Katz, B. & Miledi, R. (1965c). The effect of temperature on the synaptic delay at the neuromuscular junction. *J. Physiol.* **181,** 656.

Katz, B. & Miledi, R. (1967a). Modification of transmitter release by electrical interference with motor nerve endings. *Proc. R. Soc.* B **167,** 1.

Katz, B. & Miledi, R. (1967b). Tetrodotoxin and neuromuscular transmission. *Proc. R. Soc.* B **167,** 8.

Katz, B. & Miledi, R. (1967c). The timing of calcium action during neuromuscular transmission. *J. Physiol.* **189,** 535.

Katz, B. & Miledi, R. (1967d). A study of synaptic transmission in the absence of nerve impulses. *J. Physiol.* **192,** 407.

Keynes, R. D. (1951a). The leakage of radioactive potassium from stimulated nerve. *J. Physiol.* **113,** 99.

Keynes, R. D. (1951b). The ionic movements during nervous activity. *J. Physiol.* **114,** 119.

Keynes, R. D. (1963). Chloride in the squid giant axon. *J. Physiol.* **169,** 690.

Keynes, R. D. & Lewis, P. R. (1951a). The resting exchange of radioactive potassium in crab nerve. *J. Physiol.* **113,** 73.

Keynes, R. D. & Lewis, P. R. (1951b). The sodium and potassium content of cephalopod nerve fibres. *J. Physiol.* **114,** 151.

KOECHLIN, B. A. (1955). On the chemical composition of the axoplasm of squid giant nerve fibres with particular reference to its ion pattern. *J. biophys. biochem. Cytol.* **1,** 511.

KRNJEVIĆ, K. & MITCHELL, J. F. (1961). The release of acetylcholine in the isolated rat diaphragm. *J. Physiol.* **155,** 246.

KRNJEVIĆ, K. & VAN GELDER, N. M. (1961). Tension changes in crayfish stretch receptors. *J. Physiol.* **159,** 310.

KUFFLER, S. W. (1967). The Ferrier Lecture: Neuroglial cells: physiological properties and a potassium mediated effect of neuronal activity on the glial membrane potential. *Proc. R. Soc.* B **168,** 1.

KUFFLER, S. W. & EYZAGUIRRE, C. (1955). Synaptic inhibition in an isolated nerve cell. *J. gen. Physiol.* **39,** 155.

LILEY, A. W. (1956). The quantal components of the mammalian end-plate potential. *J. Physiol.* **133,** 571.

LINDBLOM, U. (1962). The relation between stimulus and discharge in a rapidly adapting touch receptor. *Acta physiol. scand.* **56,** 349.

LOEWENSTEIN, W. R. & MENDELSON, M. (1965). Components of receptor adaptation in a Pacinian corpuscle. *J. Physiol.* **177,** 377.

MOORE, J. W., BLAUSTEIN, M. P., ANDERSON, N. C. & NARAHASHI, T. (1967). Basis of tetrodotoxin's selectivity in blockage of squid axons. *J. gen. Physiol.* **50,** 1401.

MENDELL, L. M. & WALL, P. (1964). Presynaptic hyperpolarization: a role for fine afferent fibres. *J. Physiol.* **172,** 274.

OTSUKA, M., IVERSON, L. L., HALL, Z. W. & KRAVITZ, E. A. (1966). Release of gamma-aminobutyric acid from inhibitory nerves of lobster. *Proc. Natl. Acad. Sci. U.S.* **56,** 1110.

PITTS, R. F. (1942). Excitation and inhibition of phrenic motor neurons. *J. Neurophysiol.* **5,** 75.

ROBERTSON, J. D. (1955). Recent electron microscope observations on the ultrastructure of the crayfish median-to-motor giant synapse. *Exp. Cell Res.* **8,** 226.

ROBERTSON, J. D. (1956). The ultrastructure of a reptilian myoneural junction. *J. biophys. biochem. Cytol.* **2,** 381.

ROBERTSON, J. D. (1960). The molecular structure and contact relationship of cell membranes. *Progr. Biophys. Biophys. Chem.* **10,** 343.

ROBERTSON, J. D. (1961). Ultrastructure of excitable membranes and the crayfish median-giant synapse. *Ann. N.Y. Acad. Sci.* **94,** 339.

SHANES, A. M. & BERMAN, M. D. (1955). Kinetics of ion movement in the squid giant axon. *J. gen. Physiol.* **39,** 279.

SHOLL, D. A. (1956). *The Organisation of the Cerebral Cortex*, p. 3. Hafner, N.Y.

SMITH, T. G., WUERKER, R. B. & FRANK, K. (1967). Membrane impedance changes during synaptic transmission in cat spinal motoneurons. *J. Neurophysiol.* **30,** 1072.

TAKEUKI, A. & TAKEUKI, N. (1959). Active phase of frog's end-plate potential. *J. Neurophysiol.* **22,** 395.

TAKEUKI, A. & TAKEUKI, N. (1960). On the permeability of end-plate membrane during the action of transmitter. *J. Physiol.* **154,** 52.

TAKEUKI, A. & TAKEUKI, N. (1962). Electrical changes in pre- and postsynaptic axons of the giant synapse of Loligo. *J. gen. Physiol.* **45,** 1181.

TAKEUKI, A. & TAKEUKI, N. (1964). The effect on crayfish muscle of iontophoretically applied glutamate. *J. Physiol.* **170,** 296.

TERZUOLO, C. A. & ARAKI, T. (1961). An analysis of intra- versus extracellular potential changes associated with activity of single spinal motoneurons. *Ann. N.Y. Acad. Sci.* **94,** 547.

TERZUOLO, C. A. & WASHIZU, Y. (1962). Relation between stimulus strength, generator potential and impulse frequency in stretch receptor of Crustacea. *J. Neurophysiol.* **25,** 56.

WHITTAKER, V. P. (1964). Investigations on the storage sites of biogenic amines in the central nervous system. *Progr. Brain Res.* **8,** 90.

Index

NOTES

NOTES

NOTES

NOTES

NOTES